This book is dedicted to the patients and families that have
put their trust in me.

GIFTED: Genetic Information For Treating Eating Disorders

By Michael Lutter, MD/PHD

Published March 2023

eBook ISBN: 9798215049723

Print Book ISBN: 9798215017067

About the Author

Michael Lutter, MD/PhD is a physician-scientist who has worked in the fields of eating disorders, depression, and anxiety since 2007. Dr. Lutter graduated from the University of Chicago in 1996 with a degree in Biological Chemistry before completing the Medical Scientist Training Program at the University of Texas Southwestern Medical Center in Dallas, Texas and earning MD and PHD degrees in 2003. His interest in eating disorders began during his Psychiatry Residency Program at UT Southwestern. From 2008-2016 he ran a research program on the genetic and neurobiological basis of eating disorders at UT Southwestern Medical Center and later at the University of Iowa before transitioning to full time clinical care working at the Eating Recovery Center from 2016-202.

Dr Lutter founded Precision Psychiatry in 2019 to pursue his vision of integrating new scientific approaches into the treatment of patients with eating disorders, depression, and anxiety. Using the knowledge he gained from his years doing genetic and behavioral neuroscience research, he developed Genetic Information For Treating Eating Disorders (GIFTED).

To learn more about GIFTED and Dr Lutter visit:

www.Precision-Psychiatry.com

Acknowledgements

I would like to thank the following individuals and groups:

- Jessica Setnick, A.J. Robison, and Melissa Judd for reviewing early drafts of the manuscript.
- Aaron L. Gravely, MD for editing and proofreading of the final manuscript.
- Articulate Graphics (http://www.articulategraphics.com/) created the medical illustrations and animations in Chapter 7 (Anorexia Nervosa).
- All other illustrations were made using BioRender (https://www.biorender.com/).
- Voice acting for the animation was performed by Kim Fuller (www.kimfullervoice.com).
- Cover art was designed in Canva (https://www.canva.com/)

Contents

<u>Glossary</u>

Note: items in the glossary are <u>underlined</u> in the main text of the book

Anesthetic- *a medication used to temporarily decrease consciousness and sensation, usually for a surgical procedure*

BMI- *stands for Body Mass Index, a formula used by many health care providers to determine if a patient is underweight, normal weight, or overweight/obese. BMI is calculated by diving a person's weight by the square of their height*

Bioinformatics- *a field of science that uses computers to analyze large sets of biological data*

Cannabinoid hyperemesis syndrome- *severe nausea and vomiting that is sometimes seen in regular cannabis (marijuana) users who suddenly stop using cannabis*

Carnitine- *a molecule that helps transport long-chain fatty acids into the mitochondria to be turned into energy*

Case report- *A detailed report describing a rare or unusual occurrence in a single patient or small group of patients. Case reports are considered to be low-quality medical research*

Circadian entrainment therapy- *a behavioral therapy that uses powerful entrainers of the biological clock to regulate sleep/wake cycles and meal patterns in patients with unstable circadian rhythms*

Circadian rhythm- *any bodily process that fluctuates on a 24-hour cycle, including sleep/wake cycles, appetite, body temperature, and metabolism*

Citation- *a reference to another scientific article or book to support claims that are made*

CoQ10- *also known as coenzyme Q10 or ubiquinone-10, is a molecule made by the body that helps the mitochondria convert food into energy*

Cytokine- *a group of proteins that mainly function by sending signals between immune system cells*

Diagnostic and Statistical Manual- *a book published by the American Psychiatric Association that lists the criteria to diagnose all mental illnesses*

Effectiveness study- *a type of research study that looks at how treatments work in 'real world settings'*

Efficacy study- *a type of research study that looks at how treatments work under 'ideal settings'*

Endocannabinoids- *a system of lipid neurotransmitters in the body that send retrograde (backward) to regulate signaling of neurons, the endocannabinoid system affects a wide-range of bodily functions including mood, pain, appetite, and memory and is the target of drug cannabis (marijuana)*

Endogenous opioid system- *a system composed of several peptide neurotransmitters and their receptors that regulate many bodily processes including pain, stress responses, breathing, appetite, and digestive function, the endogenous opioid system is the target of several medications like morphine and oxycodone and drugs of abuse like heroin*

Epigenomics- *a scientific field that studies how modifications to DNA affects the expression of genes encoded by DNA*

Essential amino acid- *the nine amino acids that cannot be made by the body and are therefore essential to obtain in the diet, they are isoleucine, leucine, valine, lysine, histidine, methionine, phenylalanine, threonine, and tryptophan*

Exome- *the part of the DNA that includes the protein-encoding genes*

Expert opinion- *medical recommendations made by a group of designated experts, usually when high quality research (like randomized controlled trials) is not yet available*

Fatty acids- *are the building blocks of more complex fats or lipids, consisting of a carboxylic acid group (-COOH) attached to a chain of 4-28 hydrocarbons (-CH$_2$).*

Functional MRI- *a type of MRI scan that looks at the brain activity of a person while performing a task*

Genetic mutation- *a change in the DNA code that damages protein functioning*

Genetic variant- *a change in the DNA code that either has no effect on protein functioning or changes protein functioning in a way that is not harmful*

Genome- *all of the DNA in the chromosomes*

Genome-wide association study- *a type of genetic study that scientists use to find genetic factors that are associated with a specific disease or trait*

Gut-brain neuropeptides- *Neurotransmitters that are made from genes in the DNA and that regulate a variety of functions related to appetite, metabolism, and GI system function*

Hamwi formula- *a method for estimating ideal body weight, in women the formula is 100 lb + 5 lb for every inch in height above 5 foot tall, in men the formula is 106 lb + 6 lb for every inch in height above 5 foot tall*

Impact factor- *a statistic frequently used to measure the influence of a scientific journal, it is calculated by finding the average number of a times a scientific paper published in that journal was cited in the previous two years*

Lipidomics- *a field of biology that tries to identify and measure all of the lipids in a cell or organism*

Lipoic Acid- *a cofactor that is required for several of the chemical reactions involved in turning food into energy*

Long chain fatty acid- *a fatty acid with a hydrocarbon chain that is between 13-21 carbons long, requires carnitine and the carnitine palmitoyl transferase system in order to enter the mitochondria and be broken down into energy*

Major allele- *when there are two possible nucleotides at a certain position in the DNA, the major allele is the one that is more common in the population*

Mediobasal hypothalamus- *a region of the brain that is involved in the control of appetite, fat storage and energy expenditure*

Metabolomics- *a field of biology that tries to identify and measure all of the biological molecules in a cell or organism*

Microbiome- *all of the microorganisms living in the GI tract*

Minor allele- *when there are two possible nucleotides at a certain position in the DNA, the minor allele is the one that is less common in the population*

Mitochondria- *a part of the cell that is mainly involved in converting food into energy, but has a number of other functions including heat production, making certain molecules for the cell to use, and regulating cell death*

Monogenic- *monogenic diseases are caused by mutations in a single gene*

mTOR- *stands for either Mammalian Target Of Rapamycin (mTOR) or Mechanistic Target Of Rapamycin, it serves as one of the primary nutrient sensors in the cells of the body*

Neuropeptide- *a neurotransmitter that is made with instructions from a gene in the DNA*

Neurotransmitter- *a molecule that is released by a neuron to send a signal to another part of the body, such as a muscle, gland, or another neuron*

Number needed to harm- *the number of people who need to receive a specific medical treatment to cause one person to have a specific side effect (such as a blood clot, liver failure, or death)*

Number needed to treat- *the number of people who need to receive a specific medical treatment to prevent one person from having a bad outcome (such as a heart attack, stroke, or death).*

Peer review process- *a method for evaluating the value of a scientific work (such as a grant or paper) by using one or more people with similar expertise (peers) to judge its quality*

Polygenic- *polygenic diseases are caused by mutations in more than one gene*

Precision medicine- *or personalized medicine, is a field of study that uses information relating to a person's genes, environment, and lifestyle to create individually tailored medical treatments*

Private mutation- *a rare or novel gene mutation that is usually found only in a single person or family*

Proteomics- *a field of biology that tries to identify and measure all of the proteins in a cell or organism*

Psychoactive- *a drug or medication that alters one's thoughts, perceptions, mood, consciousness, or behavior.*

Psychoanalytic psychotherapy- *or psychoanalysis is a method of exploring the unconscious impulses using techniques such as dream interpretation, free association, and analysis of resistance to change*

Psychopharmacology- *a field of study examining psychoactive substances*

Randomized controlled trial- *a type of research study in which individuals are randomly assigned to a treatment (the experimental group) or a placebo (the control group)*

Recovered- *when a patient no longer has any symptoms after receiving a specific treatment*

Responded- *when a patient's symptoms have decreased by more than 50% after a treatment but are still present*

Satiation- *refers to how long a person feels full or satisfied after a meal, satiation controls when a person is hungry again after eating*

Satiety- *refers to feelings of fullness or satisfaction during a meal, satiety controls how much a person eats during a meal*

Signs- *outward manifestations of a psychiatric illness, such as bizarre behavior or talking very quickly*

Single-blinded- *the peer review process is said to be single-blinded if the reviewers know the identity of the author, but author is not aware of the identities of the reviewers, a work is double-blinded if neither side is aware of the other's identity, and unblinded if both side know the identities of the other*

SPECT- *or Single-Photon Emission Computed Tomography, is a brain imaging technique that uses small amounts of a radioactive compound to measure brain activity of an awake person*

Symptoms- *manifestations of a psychiatric illness that only a person experiences, such as intrusive thoughts or hallucinations*

Tetrahydrobiopterin- *a molecule made by the body that is required for the synthesis of several neurotransmitters including serotonin, dopamine, norepinephrine, and melatonin*

Transcription factor- *a protein that controls the a certain set of genes are turned on or turned off*

Transcriptomics- *a field of biology that tries to identify and measure all of the mRNA molecules in a cell or organism*

Triglycerides- *a type of fat composed of three fatty acids linked together by a glycerol molecule, primarily used as a way to store energy for later use*

Vitamin B- *a group of water-soluble vitamins that play important roles in metabolism, especially in processes related to turning food into energy, patients with anorexia are more likely to have mutations in gene related to*

- *Thiamine (B1)*
- *Niacin (B3)*

- *Panthothenic acid (B5)*
- *Pyridoxine (B6)*
- *Biotin (B7)*
- *Folate (B9)*
- *Cobalamin (B12)*

Vitamin D- *a vitamin that can either be produced by the skin in response to sunlight or obtained in the diet, vitamin D is a key regulator of calcium and phosphorus levels in the body*

Waitlist control group- *in a research study, a waitlist control group is a group of participants that is randomly selected to wait to receive the experimental treatment (instead of receiving the placebo treatment) and serves the comparison group*

Whole exome sequencing- *a type of DNA sequencing that only analyzes the DNA around the protein-coding genes*

Prologue: "Something Better"

In 2005, I was about half-way through my residency in psychiatry. Two years earlier I had graduated from the Medical Scientist Training Program at the University of Texas Southwestern Medical School with two doctoral degrees: a Medical Doctorate and a Doctorate in Philosophy (PhD) in Integrative Biology. My goal at the time was to pursue a career as a physician-scientist. The idea was that I would see patients as a medical doctor and then use the knowledge I gained from these interactions to better inform the scientific research I conducted in my laboratory. In the ideal scenario, I would discover some great new treatment that I could then bring to my patients.

I decided to become a psychiatrist for two reasons. First, I thought, of all the fields of medicine, psychiatry had the most interesting unanswered questions. How are memories formed? What causes paranoia or a hallucination? Why are some people not able to stop using drugs or alcohol despite the consequences? Why do some people believe they are too fat when they are clearly starving themselves? I could think of nothing better than a life spent trying to answer these questions while helping people in the process. The second reason why I chose psychiatry is far less idealistic. In medical school, I was advised that you wanted to either 'be at the beginning of a field or the end of the field', meaning it was best to either be known as the first person to study a disease or as the person who developed the ultimate treatment for it. Even then, as a medical student, it was clear to me that the field of psychiatry was decades behind the rest of medicine. It felt like there was so much more to be done in psychiatry compared to everything else, and that it would be easier to make a contribution.

So here I was in 2005 meeting with one of my advisors. At the time, I was complaining about learning Freudian <u>psychoanalysis</u>, which is still in practice to this day. My advisor was a neuroscientist as well, so I asked him why he was not a more vocal critic of psychoanalysis as I knew he shared my skepticism of the field. His response was that criticism by itself is not interesting to most people unless you have "something better" to offer them. He had focused his career on trying to find a better understanding of mental illness and better treatments by using neuroscience, and he felt this was a far better use of his time than simply complaining about the *status quo*.

I have used this advice to guide my career ever since that day. This book represents the culmination of my efforts to find "something better" to offer people who are struggling with mental illness. In many ways, this book also reflects the unusual meandering path that my career has taken. The early chapters will discuss my experience doing research in academic medical centers, while the middle chapters will reflect on my time treating patients in a for-profit treatment program. The final chapters of the book will take the lessons I have learned from both experiences and present my vision for the future of psychiatry. I have tried to temper my criticism of psychiatry, as this book is meant to inspire hope, not contempt. Nonetheless some level of critique was necessary to adequately show how my frustration with the current system inspired me to find "something better."

Chapter 1: Chest Pain Syndrome

In this first chapter, I present the concept of a syndromic illness. Syndromes are a group of symptoms that usually occur together, but for which there is no known cause. Syndromes are different from diseases for which there is a well-defined cause, often with specific diagnostic tests and treatments. Psychiatry remains the one field of medicine composed almost entirely of syndromes.

Imagine walking into a doctor's office with chest pain. The doctor proceeds to ask you a series of questions about your symptoms. What things does the pain prevent you from doing? Is your heart rate faster or slower than normal? Is your temperature higher or lower? Is your breathing faster or slower? Does the pain make it difficult to sleep or are you sleeping more because you are too tired?

After questioning you, the doctor determines that you have Chest Pain Syndrome, prescribes you a pain medication, and tells you to return in a month. You come back a month later and you still have the pain in your chest, so the doctor increases the dose and has you come back a month later. You return and the pain is no better, so this time he changes your prescription to a different pain medication. After another month without improvement in your symptoms, he adds a second pain medication that works slightly differently, so now you are taking two medications for your chest pain.

After four months of no improvement (assuming you are still alive) the doctor is baffled. "I'm not sure why this isn't working? About one third of people with Chest Pain Syndrome get better after one of these medications", they tell you. At this point, the doctor gives you a few more options: Try another pain medication, make some lifestyle changes, or receive electrical stimulation on the area.

The description of this scenario might make you think that it takes place 100 years ago. Today, if you walk into a medical office with chest pain there is an extensive array of tests and procedures that can precisely determine the cause of the pain and identify the right treatment. Doctors call this process a 'work-up,' and it is important to not only receive proper treatment, but also to avoid the trial-and-error process of trying multiple treatments since receiving the wrong treatment costs time and money, exposes you to the risk of side effects, and, in the worst-case scenario, can make your symptoms worse instead of better.

In the case of chest pain, a medical work-up tries to determine if it is caused by a heart attack (lack of blood supply to the muscle of the heart), pneumonia (viral or bacterial infection of the lungs), pulmonary embolism (blood clot to the lung), aortic dissection (tear in the wall of the major blood vessel leaving the heart), pleural effusions (fluid on the lining of the lungs), or a tension pneumothorax (a tiny hole in the chest wall that allows air to get trapped between the lung and the chest wall). Each of these causes is medically addressed by a distinct treatment that directly targets the cause of the chest pain, resulting in relief of the symptoms. Such medical workups are standard in most fields, but this approach does not currently exist for psychiatry.

As crazy and imprecise as this seems, this trial-and-error approach is a pretty close approximation of the current state of psychiatry. All the major psychiatric diagnoses remain syndromes, which means that instead of using tests to diagnose a disease, we use checklists of symptoms reported by the patient and signs observed by family members or clinicians. Major depressive disorder (or major depression) is a good example of this problem. Major depression is a common problem affecting 15-20% of people in their lifetime and as many as 5% of people are chronically depressed globally. Major depression is considered the number one cause of lost days of productive life in the world and is a major factor contributing to suicide, which is one of the top 10 causes of death annually[1].

In order to be diagnosed with major depression, you need to have one "mood symptom" (feeling either sad or irritable), plus four of the remaining eight symptoms listed in the diagnostic criteria. These symptoms include lack of motivation, difficulty concentrating or making decisions, lack of energy, changes in physical activity, changes in appetite, changes in sleep, feelings of excessive guilt or worthlessness, and suicidal thoughts. Three of the criteria for major depression can change in either direction. Take physical activity, for example. In order to meet the physical activity criteria of major depression, you can either feel restless like you can't sit still or feel slow like you are stuck in mud. For appetite, you can either have no appetite and lose weight, or you can have increased appetite and gain weight. For sleep, you can either have trouble falling or staying asleep, or sleep too much.

When I was going through medical school and psychiatric residency, this discrepancy really bothered me. I knew enough about the neurobiology of sleep and appetite to know that lack of sleep/appetite are completely different processes in the brain than increased sleep/appetite. Yet, within the field of psychiatry, this contradiction is not a problem at all. Consider the case of two patients both diagnosed with major depression: The first person could be sad and not enjoy anything, have no energy, sleep all day, not take showers, change clothes, or brush their teeth for days, and feel like their arms and legs are heavy and difficult to move. The second person could report symptoms of feeling irritable and easily angered, restless like they can't sit still, not be able to sleep, and have no appetite. According to the current psychiatric diagnostic guidelines, they both have the same diagnosis of major depression, even though they *don't have a single symptom in common*.

Without knowing the cause of psychiatric disorders, prescribed treatments are bound to be imprecise. Almost all the current treatments for psychiatric disorders were discovered by chance observation and are used in a process very close to trial and error. A one in three recovery rate after treatment seems low for most fields of medicine (it certainly would not be tolerated for patients presenting to the emergency department with chest pain), but is common for the treatment of depression, psychosis, and substance abuse. In the example above of the two depressed patients, both would qualify for the exact same set of treatments, working through each treatment stepwise until one medication (or combination of medications) is found to be effective. Similar protocols exist for anxiety disorders, bipolar disorder, and schizophrenia.

But how did psychiatry get to this point? Other fields of medicine have syndromes as diagnoses, like chronic fatigue syndrome or irritable bowel syndrome, but these tend to the exception. Psychiatry, however, is composed almost entirely of syndromic diagnoses. That is, we have no objective ways of identifying the cause of psychiatric symptoms, and almost no rational treatments. We know that psychiatric illnesses are a combination of genetic risk inherited from your parents and environmental stressors, but so far, we have had little success untangling the complex relationship between how mutations in your DNA interact with your life experiences to produce symptoms of sadness, worry, hallucination, persistent drug and alcohol abuse, compulsive hand-washing, or a fear of eating. In the coming chapters, I will present my theory that psychiatric researchers have historically made the wrong assumptions on how genetic variations increase the risk of mental illness, and that entrenched institutions have discouraged the field from shifting to new approaches. Additionally, I will present examples of better ways to diagnose and treat patients and discuss what must be done to truly revolutionize the field of psychiatry.

Chapter 2: The Stakeholders

To understand why psychiatry has fallen so far behind other fields of medicine, it helps to first identify and understand the major stakeholders and their incentives. In Chapter 2, I will discuss the groups and organizations that have a major stake in the field of mental health.

<u>American Psychiatric Association</u>

The American Psychiatric Association is the professional organization that represents the interests of Psychiatrists. The American Psychiatric Association has an interesting auxiliary responsibility in advocating for their members. They also decide which criteria are used to diagnose mental illness. The American Psychiatric Association fulfills this responsibility by publishing a book called the Diagnostic and Statistical Manual, of which we are now on the 5th edition (referred to commonly as DSM-V).

The first edition of the Diagnostic and Statistical Manual was published in 1952[2]. Psychiatry was a much different field at the time. In the 1950s, over 500,000 patients per year in the United States were long-term residents of state and county psychiatric hospitals. Patients were sent to these facilities for months or even years at a time to be housed and, hopefully, treated[3]. Diagnosis of mental illness was highly variable at the time in part because the diagnostic criteria were vague, open to interpretation, and not standardized.

The most prominent psychiatrists of the time were disciples of Sigmund Freud. Freudian psychiatrists practice <u>psychoanalysis</u> and believe that the root of psychiatric illness lay in subconscious, internal conflicts of which the patient is unaware. True diagnosis depends on a psychiatrist interpreting how these conflicts develop over time. In the first and second editions of the Diagnostic and Statistical Manual, diagnoses were based largely on these Freudian interpretations and, as such, were difficult to objectively measure[4]. The first two editions were largely an academic exercise without much impact on the day-to-day practice of psychiatry.

The third edition of the Diagnostic and Statistical Manual, published in 1980, marked a major change that arguably ushered in the current era of psychiatry[5]. The Diagnostic and Statistical Manual-III shifted away from subjective interpretations of patients' thoughts and focused more on objective criteria that could be clinically observed. 'Symptoms' are things that patients report, like feeling sad or tired. 'Signs' are things that can be witnessed by people like family members or clinicians, such as restless pacing or bizarre/disorganized behaviors.

Once the Diagnostic and Statistical Manual-III allowed for diagnosis, the next step was to use it for patient care. As managed care began to sweep through the United States, the Diagnostic and Statistical Manual-III criteria became the basis for deciding who was eligible to get treatment and which treatments would be available. Small differences in wording or the interpretation of the wording could decide who did and did not qualify for treatment and swing billions of dollars in health care spending. The incentives were clear to anyone supplying mental health care— broader, more inclusive criteria were more lucrative, because they reached the most people. The American Psychiatric Association has followed up with publication of the fourth and fifth editions of the Diagnostic and Statistical Manual, each larger than the one before (Chart 1) [6]. The total number of diagnoses and the number of people affected has continued to increase. It is now estimated that close to half of the population in the United States meets criteria for one of the almost 300 diagnoses in the Diagnostic and Statistical Manual-V[7].

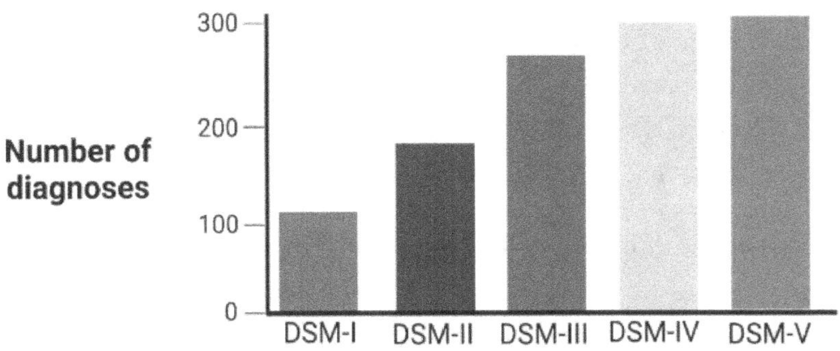

<u>National Institute of Health (NIH)</u>

The National Institute of Health is primarily responsible for conducting research to improve the diagnosis, prevention, and treatment of illness. The National Institute of Health is separated into multiple smaller institutes, each with a distinct role. Several of these institutes are relevant to psychiatry, including the National Institute of Mental Health (NIMH), the National Institute of Drug Abuse (NIDA), and the National Institute of Alcohol Abuse and Alcoholism (NIAAA)[8].

The individual institutes of the National Institute of Health support research in two ways. Each institute keeps a small percentage of their budget to conduct their own internal research projects (commonly called intramural research). But the primary role of the individual institutes is to dole out money for research in the form of grants (extramural research). Individual researchers can apply for a grant from the National Institute of Health, but most grant recipients are large research universities and non-profit organizations. A researcher can request money to study anything that they feel could be important to the diagnosis, treatment, or prevention of a psychiatric illness. This type of grant is called an Investigator Initiated Study. Individual institutes like the National Institute of Mental Health can also set aside pots of money to research specific topics that they feel are important, like suicide prevention. These grants are called request for applications (or RFAs) and allow the National Institute of Health to prioritize certain areas that they feel are especially important but understudied.

Grant applications are evaluated by fellow scientists and given a score (lower scores are better like in golf). The institutions use these scores to then decide which projects to fund. Grants range in value from tens of thousands of dollars to millions of dollars. The overall budget of the National Institute of Health for 2022 was $45 billion dollars, with the National Institute of Mental Health receiving $2.213 billion, the National Institute of Drug Abuse receiving $1.853 billion, and National Institute of Alcohol Abuse and Alcoholism receiving $507.2 million.

NIH-funded research can influence patient care in many ways. For starters, the National Institute of Health can directly fund clinical trials to identify new treatments for a specific diagnosis. For example, this could occur when a researcher develops a new form of psychotherapy that improves symptoms for a condition, like generalized anxiety disorder or major depressive disorder. It might also occur when a researcher finds that a medication already used to treat a different condition in humans also helps treat the symptoms of a psychiatric illness. A good example of this is when the blood pressure medication propranolol was found to reduce symptoms of performance anxiety[9]. The National Institute of Health also funds basic science research with the goal of understanding how the human body works without necessarily having relevance to a specific disorder. For instance, the National Institute of Health funds research in worms (*C. elegans*), fruit flies (*D. melanogaster*), mice (*M. musculus*) and rats (*R. norvegicus*) to understand how neurons work, with the hope that the knowledge gained will later be relevant to human disorders. The third category is called translational research and bridges basic and clinical research. Translational research tries to use discoveries from basic science to develop novel ways to diagnose or treat psychiatric disorders.

<u>Pharmaceutical Companies</u>

Psychiatric illness is in theory a lucrative market for drug development. Psychiatric illnesses are common, disproportionately affect younger individuals, and are often chronic. This all adds up to a potentially large group of individuals who will take medications for years if not decades.

However, developing medications to treat psychiatric illness also has several unique limitations. While certain organs like the heart, lungs, liver, and kidneys are similar between humans and laboratory animals like mice and rats, the brain is distinctly different. It is impossible to ask a mouse whether it is hallucinating or is feeling paranoid. Likewise, it is difficult to model higher cognitive processes like hopelessness or suicidal ideation in a mouse.

After the initial success of antidepressant medications like Prozac (fluoxetine) and antipsychotic/mood stabilizing medications like Risperdal (risperidone), pharmaceutical companies poured millions of dollars into research programs to identify new medications. Those efforts have largely failed to lead to the development of new medicines and the research and development programs have been mostly shut down[10]. Most of the recently approved medications in psychiatry are minor changes to older drugs, and deemed 'me-too' drugs, because of their close resemblance to previous medications[11]. While many of these follow-up drugs have potential advantages over older medications (usually reducing unwanted side effects like weight gain or sexual dysfunction), they are not required to be more effective, less expensive, or safer than their older counterparts. In order to get approved by the Food and Drug Administration, a medication need only show that it is better than placebo.

One hope is that by heavily investing in basic and translational research, the National Institute of Health will encourage private companies to find new treatments. Developing a new medication is a long and expensive process. The National Institute of Health hopes that private companies will use the knowledge produced by the basic science research that it funds to identify potential new treatments. This plan, however, depends on National Institute of Health-funded researchers, pharmaceutical companies, the American Psychiatric Association, and the Food and Drug Administration all agreeing on the same criteria for what constitutes an illness.

<u>Treatment Providers</u>

If the role of academic researchers and pharmaceutical companies is to develop new treatments for mental illness, then it is the responsibility of the treatment providers to deliver that care to patients. The term 'treatment provider' covers a broad array of medical professionals. Psychiatrists specialize in <u>psychopharmacology</u> (the use of medications to treat mental illness), but most psychiatric medications are prescribed by other medical specialists (such as family medicine, pediatrics, internal medicine, gynecology, and neurology), psychiatric nurse practitioners, psychiatric pharmacists, and (in five states) psychologists. Psychologists traditionally are highly trained in delivering psychotherapy (also known as talk therapy), but many other clinicians provide psychotherapy services as well, including social workers, licensed professional counselors, licensed marital and family therapists, and some psychiatrists. Many other medical professionals also participate in the treatment of psychiatric patients, including nurses, social workers, dietitians, speech and language therapists, physical therapists, occupational therapists, and behavioral health technicians. Outside of the medical profession, there are many other groups and individuals who provide both paid and volunteer services that can help in the treatment of patients with mental illness, including coaching and life development services, complementary medicine, and sobriety programs like Alcoholics Anonymous (AA).

The job of a treatment provider is two-fold. They must provide effective treatments, but they also have to run a successful business. Unfortunately, these two goals can sometimes be in conflict. Treatment (prescribing medication, performing psychotherapy, providing nutrition advice, etc.) is paid for by either medical insurance or through cash payment. Most treatments in psychiatry are provided face to face and require significant investments of time. Many times, the only way to increase profitability is to decrease the amount of time spent with a patient or to provide treatment in a group setting. I know of psychiatry practices that expect their providers to see 4-5 patients *per hour*. Once you factor in things like paperwork, that leaves less than 10 minutes of talking to the patient. Likewise, many psychiatric hospitals and treatment programs provide most of their care through group psychotherapy, in which patients with different diagnoses all receive the same treatment. Thus, the need to stay afloat financially can often prevent providers from delivering the most effective treatment to each patient individually.

<u>Patient Advocacy Groups</u>

While clinicians, researchers, and private companies all have their own incentives (which mostly align with profit and recognition), the interests of the patients can often be secondary. Patient advocacy groups fill this role by giving voice to the thoughts and feelings of patients and their families. Other areas of medicine have very well-established and powerful groups like the American Heart

Association, the American Cancer Association, and the American Diabetes Association, which are able to shape public policy.

There are many groups that advocate for patients with mental illness, including the National Association for Mental Illness (NAMI) and various groups that represent subsets of patients such as autism, eating disorders, and Alzheimer's disease. I sympathize the most with these groups, as they are sincerely trying to improve the lives of patients while often working against the entrenched interests of the other groups.

In theory, these groups all have their different roles and should be able to work together to advance that cause of mental illness. The reality, I find, is that while patient advocacy groups do engage with all the relevant groups, there is very little positive interaction between the other groups who tend to work independently toward their own agendas.

Chapter 3: How Research Works

Scientists pride themselves on the rigor of the scientific method, which is supposed to identify knowledge without bias. While this is a worthy ideal to live up to, the truth is that most scientists are influenced either consciously or unconsciously by the incentives that shape their work. In Chapter 3, I will describe the biomedical research complex at major universities and academic medical centers and discuss how lack of oversight has fueled an epidemic of bad science.

<u>University Researchers</u>

Most National Institute of Health-funded research is conducted at academic medical centers and research universities. Each institution is usually organized into departments. Medical schools are often organized around established medical specialties like surgery, pediatrics, pathology, radiology, neurology, or psychiatry. Basic science departments will often form around areas of common interest like neuroscience, genetics, or biochemistry. Each department is headed by a chair and staffed by a series of scientists. At medical schools or universities, these scientists are usually called a professor (ranking from Associate to Assistant to Full Professors as their careers develop). Each individual professor has their own independent research program. A professor has the option to choose to research whatever they think is interesting or important, but they are also responsible for obtaining the funding to pay for the research, and this is not cheap. Even small research laboratories of new Assistant Professors can cost hundreds of thousands of dollars to operate per year. Large laboratories of established Full Professors might spend millions of dollars per year.

Some of the funding comes from teaching students or from patient care (if it is a clinical department that also treats patients). Departments at major universities also have endowments created with money given by wealthy donors. These endowments stay in investment funds, but some of the returns from the investments can be used each year for research. Each individual professor is then responsible for writing grant proposals to get funding to cover the remaining cost of doing research. The National Institute of Health is the most common source for funding, and obtaining continuous funding from the National Institute of Health is considered essential to establishing your credibility as an academic scientist. Each grant application is dozens of pages long and includes sections to describe the importance of the work, the design of the experiments, and how the data will be analyzed, as well as sections to highlight the researcher's qualifications, the safety of the research space, and a budget plan explaining how the money will be spent.

A typical National Institute of Health grant application can take weeks to months to prepare and submit. After a grant is submitted, it then goes through a rigorous review process, which can take several months to complete, and then more time to find out if the grant is funded, and then even more time to receive the money in an account that can be used to pay for research. Most grant applications sent to the National Institute of Health are reviewed by the Center for Scientific Review[12] and are sent to something called a study section, which consists of a group of scientists with an expertise in certain topics like Molecular Neurogenetics (MNG) or Psychosocial Development, Risk, and Prevention (PDRP). The entire grant application is then read by three scientists on the study section who give out a preliminary score. After the grant is thoroughly read by these three individuals, all the members of the study section then meet, and each grant is presented and critiqued by everyone on the committee before it receives a final score.

After a grant proposal receives a score, it then returns to the original institute (like the National Institute of Mental Health of the National

Institute of Drug Addiction), where the scientists called program officers decide which grants to fund. Program officers make their decision based largely upon the scores that the grants receive, but they do have some discretion to fund areas of research that their institute feels is important but underrepresented.

In my personal experience, the program officers of the National Institute of Mental Health were unquestionably the least qualified and least successful group of scientists I ever had to work with. I think most people who have a loved one struggling with a mental illness would be shocked to realize that the only exposure that many program officers get to the illnesses that they oversee researching comes from reading articles and attending conferences. The program officer's performance is judged by the research output of the grants they fund (their "portfolio"), and the key factor there is the number of scientific papers that result from the grant and the popularity of the journals in which those papers are published (more on this later). I find that most program officers are completely out of touch with answering scientific questions that are relevant to clinicians, and instead focus on funding the research that is most likely to get into top journals (and advance their own careers).

After all of this, only about 20% of grants submitted to the National Institute of Health are funded, although for certain types of grants the funding rate can drop below 10%[13]. So, what happens to the scientists who don't get funded the first time they submit a grant? A scientist can take the feedback they have received on the study section of their grant proposal, make the suggested changes, and then send it back to be reviewed again, hoping that it gets a better score the second time around. It obviously takes less time to edit a grant proposal that is already written than it does to write a new grant entirely from scratch, but it is still a considerable drain on the researcher's time. In most cases, the National Institute of Health only reviews grant proposal three times a year, and it takes several months for a grant to be reviewed, scored, and accepted or rejected for funding. As a result, most researchers find themselves in a cycle every few months of writing grants, then teaching and doing research while waiting for the grant to get reviewed, and then writing (or re-writing) a grant again, and then doing research and teaching again until a project is eventually funded (or not).

While National Institute of Health funding is the largest source of funding for psychiatric research, there are other organizations that contribute to scientific research funding as well. Some of these organizations include patient advocacy groups, pharmaceutical companies, and private donors. These grants are typically smaller in the amount of funding that they provide, but often are either easier to write or easier to obtain because more than 20% of the grants are funded. National Institute of Health grants that are not funded can often be used as a starting point for writing one of these grants as well, which also makes the process easier. These types of grants can be a nice way to smooth out the boom or bust nature of the National Institute of Health grant cycle.

In addition to the money that Professors bring in to directly support their own research (called 'direct' funds), each grant also comes with additional money to support the infrastructure of the institution that the researcher works at (called 'indirect' funds). In theory, this money is used to pay for things like maintenance, water, and electricity in the research buildings, but it is also used to support things like safety monitoring and libraries. Unlike 'direct' funds that pay for research and require clear budgets, university administrators have broad discretion on how to use 'indirect' funds to support research. As you can imagine, university officials aggressively seek out scientists with large amounts of grant funding to get 'indirect' funds for their own pet projects. This quirk of the funding system incentivizes universities to seek out the scientists with the largest grants even if they have questionable reputations and is another way in which the current system enables questionable scientific research.

Conducting Research

In theory, a researcher is not supposed to conduct the research until it is funded. In practice, however, most researchers have already started the project before obtaining funding (at least this was my experience in basic and translational research). When a grant is received, the funds are more often used to finish the work the grant was written to do and then begin a new project that will be used for the next grant application. Most of the actual research in universities is carried out by a combination of students and technicians. Students are either in graduate school, working toward a doctorate degree, or they are postdoctoral fellows, meaning they have already earned their doctorate degree and they are getting more experience with the intention of getting a job as an Assistant Professor somewhere else. Technicians are typically either high school or college graduates who are working in the lab as a job and not as a student or trainee. Most Professors put graduate students and postdoctoral fellows in charge of projects because they are highly motivated and don't have the same work hour restrictions that a technician would as an employee. It is not uncommon for Professors to assign projects to students that require working 7 days a week for months at a time.

The Peer Review Process

Once the data are collected and analyzed, it is time to write the paper summarizing the project and its findings. Scientific papers (and to a lesser extent patents) are the primary output of research scientists. A paper is supposed to tell a complete scientific story. It is not enough to find some interesting results and just put them out there for the world to see. In theory, a paper is supposed to follow the scientific method.

That is, a scientist is supposed to present an important question that remains unanswered, predict what the correct answer is (the hypothesis), and then show how their research either supports the hypothesis or suggests that the hypothesis is incorrect and should be rejected. In practice, most basic scientists are taught to write papers 'backwards. In other words, they start with the data they collected and then work retroactively to make a hypothesis that is supported by the data they already have. This makes for clearer reading and makes a paper more likely to be published by a top journal.

Papers are long and can also take weeks or months to write like a grant application. They typically include an 'introduction' section giving background information, a 'methods' section which is supposed to describe how the experiments were performed with enough detail for another scientist to replicate the work, a 'results' section where findings are presented, a 'discussion' section where the meaning of the findings are interpreted, and finally the 'bibliography' along with the actual data, usually in the form of graphs and tables.

Once a scientific paper is put together, the manuscript is then submitted to a scientific journal for review. In theory, the journal is only supposed to determine the quality of the work by conducting an anonymous review of the paper by fellow scientists, the so-called 'peer review process'. An Editor for the journal will screen the papers that are submitted and decide which ones are worthy of going out to be peer reviewed. They will then contact two to five scientists with expertise in the topic to read over the paper and provide feedback. The process is considered 'single-blinded' in that the reviewers know the identity of the authors of the papers, but the authors do not know who reviewed their paper. This anonymity is supposed to allow reviewers to be honest in their critiques without fear of retaliation, but in practice it is often weaponized against the author of the paper. I have known reviewers that have rejected or delayed the work of competitors, because they had similar results that they were trying to publish first. On the other hand, if a reviewer does like a paper, it is not uncommon to use that as leverage for future benefits. It is very common for other scientists to tell a colleague they gave them a favorable review when they meet in person at a conference. The person who gave a good review will then request this colleague as a reviewer for their own papers or grants hoping for a favorable review in return. While this practice is not technically illegal, I am aware of actual *quid pro quo* agreements between pairs of scientists or small groups of scientists to always give one another good reviews on grants and papers.

Once the two to five reviewers have returned their critiques, the Editor of the journal will then decide the fate of the paper. The Editor can decide either to:

1. Accept the paper (usually with just changes to the text),
2. Send it back to the author for additional experiments, or
3. Reject it outright.

Straight up acceptance of a paper without new experiments is uncommon. The culture of the research community is to send papers back for more research. Many scientists feel they have failed their duty as a reviewer if they don't suggest additional experiments. The author can then decide whether to do the experiments that the Editor requests and include the results in a revised manuscript or to just pull the paper and submit it again to a new journal. In practice, most scientists try to perform the suggested experiments and then include the new results in a revised manuscript, but this can come at great cost. Top end journals can send a paper back to the author for several rounds of revisions before finally accepting it for publication, which can take months or years and be quite expensive. It also incentivizes scientific fraud. In my time doing research, I was aware of probably around ten instances of flat-out data fabrication that occurred in the laboratories of my colleagues. About half of those cases came when a graduate student or postdoctoral fellow was doing experiments suggested by an Editor during the review process. It turns out that when an Editor tells a researcher they need a specific finding to get the paper accepted at a top journal, some researchers will get that result any way that they can.

<u>Getting Published</u>

Once a paper has been accepted for publication, the researcher now has a choice to make: They can either choose to let the paper be published as 'open access', or not. Open access journals allow the work to become freely available to the public immediately, but the author usually must pay several thousands of dollars for this privilege. Alternatively, the author can publish for free in certain journals, but in doing so they agree to hand over the rights to their work to the journal for a certain period of time. The journal then sells access to the research published in the journals back to scientists by charging subscription fees to libraries and pharmaceutical companies. So, in essence, research that has been funded by the government or private donors and peer-reviewed by fellow scientists for free is then published either: 1) as available for everyone to see for an upfront 'open-access' fee or 2) for free but with access limited to those who pay for it.

The fees to access journal articles are not cheap, either. A single article in a top journal like Nature is $32 (as of January of 2023), while an annual subscription is $199. And that is for just one journal! Large university systems pay millions of dollars per year to access research that they have freely handed over to the journals[14]. The current system would be the equivalent of the government (or a not-for-profit organization) paying someone to write a book, the content of the book being fact-checked for free by a colleague, and then handed over to a book publisher who turns around and charges everyone to buy the book. If this sounds like a lucrative business model, that is because it is. Profit margins for academic publishers can be as high as 40%[15], which places it among the most profitable industries in the world[16].

<u>Citations</u>

The bibliography of a scientific paper may seem like the least important section, but it is strangely critical. The author is supposed to cite the work of other scientists if it is important to the understanding or interpretation of the paper. For example, I wrote a paper where we reported a genetic mutation that increases the risk of developing anorexia nervosa. In that paper, we noted that the protein produced by this gene is found in areas of the brain thought to be relevant to the development of anorexia[17] (called the anterior cingulate cortex and insular cortex), which supported our theory that this mutation could increase the risk of developing anorexia by disrupting the function of the anterior cingulate cortex and insular cortex. As I was not the person who first identified that the function of these brain regions is altered in patients with anorexia, I then 'cited' the paper that reported this finding to provide support for my statement. <u>Citations</u> are supposed to be used for any statement that is not considered common knowledge. Citations have become a proxy for the quality of a paper. A paper is considered influential if a lot of other papers cite it in their bibliography. Papers that are frequently cited in other papers are considered to be higher quality. The goal of a scientist is to have their work cited by other scientists as much as possible.

Scientific journals in turn are also ranked based upon the number of citations that each of the papers that they publish receive as well. A popular method of ranking scientific journals is via their <u>Impact Factor</u>, which is the average number of times that a paper within the previous two years has been cited in the current year. For instance, a top-tier journal like the New England Journal of Medicine had an impact factor of 91.12 in 2020. Put a different way, the average paper published in the

New England Journal of Medicine in either 2018 or 2019 was cited in the bibliographies of other papers 91.12 times in 2020. For the sake of comparison, less prestigious journals have an impact factor in the single digits.

It does not take a very close examination to realize that the current system is not very good at rewarding quality research and is often easily gamed. The most obvious flaw is that all citations are treated equally, so even if a paper is referenced for being wrong, it still gets counted as a citation. In fact, one analysis found that many of the most highly cited papers are "probably wrong"[18].

Beyond this obvious flaw, there are other ways that journals and individual scientists can manipulate their citations. The most obvious is by referencing their own papers, a term called self-citation. While some level of self-citation is probably inevitable, it can be taken to extremes. For example, instead of simply writing out how an experiment was performed in the 'methods' section, many authors will self-cite their previous publications that used similar methods. I can remember one instance in which the paper I was reading, rather than describing the method, cited work from a previous paper, which in turn cited work from a previous paper, and I ultimately had to go back seven papers to find a description of the original method used to perform an experiment that was originally published in the 1950s.

One study found that the median self-citation rate was 12.7%, or about one out of every eight references in a paper is to the author's own work, with over 250 scientists citing their own work in 50% of their references[19]. Other forms of manipulation are much harder to detect. A common practice that I noted when I was still submitting research papers was to cite papers of people likely to be reviewers in order to garner their favor. A more unscrupulous method is to use the anonymous peer-review system to force people to cite their papers. I have known anonymous reviewers who have required authors to cite certain papers that the reviewer wrote as a condition of accepting a paper for publication.

Journals likewise have strong incentives to increase their impact factors to rise in the rankings list. Many journals have been criticized for being more likely to publish papers with highly controversial conclusions, which are more likely to be cited, but also more likely to be wrong[20]. In my personal experience, I have seen several instances in which Editors 'suggested' experiments to authors that would make the paper more likely to be accepted. Most of these 'suggestions' were for very high-risk experiments that were unlikely to be real but would greatly elevate interest in the paper by making splashy conclusions that would get more citations.

Many journals are reluctant to publish articles that are less likely to be cited, like original research on rare diseases. Instead, some journals will choose to publish things like review articles, which are papers that summarize the findings of several original research papers but don't include any new research. A review article would be equivalent to a journalist writing a year-end summary of all the major news events and including links to all the original news stories without doing any new reporting. Review articles are popular to write for a few reasons. Firstly, an author can reference their own papers, which gives them extra citations. Secondly, a thorough review article can summarize over a hundred papers. For this reason, review articles are often used as a reference by later papers so that the authors can point to one summary instead of citing each individual original paper separately. In this way, one can 'steal' citations from papers of competitors and replace them with citations to their own review article.

There is one additional way that scientists can game the system to get additional citations for their work. Decades ago, a paper may only have one or two authors (usually the Professor and the student) making it easy to attribute credit for the work. If you were an author on a paper, it meant that you really contributed a lot to the work that went into publishing it. Now, basic science research will often have over 10 authors, and many genetic and clinical papers will have dozens of authors. Scientists have devised weird quirks for deciding what order people are listed on the author list. In basic science, the first author on the list is typically the student (or technician) that physically did the work, while the final author (also called the corresponding author) is typically the professor who designed the experiments and wrote the grant to get the money to pay for the work. Additional students (or technicians) are then added on second to the first author, third to the first author, and so on. Professors who may have aided with the research (by providing some assistance in doing one of the experiments in the paper or providing critical reagents or animals that only their lab has access to) are typically added on the Author list second from last, third from last, and so on. Clinical researchers have their own set of rules for author placement. Clinical researchers tend to put the senior Professor first on the list, followed by other Professors, and then students and employees (maybe because students are less involved in clinical research which requires interaction with patients). In both cases, there is a secret code that represents importance on the totem pole of the author list.

<u>Accountability</u>

A key feature of the scientific method is accountability. In order to publish in a top journal, a scientist is supposed to give enough detail on how an experiment was done for any other scientist in their field to reproduce the results. Incorrect, flawed, or faked research is supposed to be exposed and rooted out by other scientists in the field so that eventually only true knowledge is left. While in theory this makes sense, in practice there is little reward for anyone to take on this policing role. Let's look at the incentives for each party:

Fellow scientists— Researchers frequently repeat the experiments of colleagues to make sure a result is true before following up on the work in their own laboratory. For example, when I was doing research, another researcher published a paper reporting that an appetite suppressing hormone also had antidepressant effects in mice[21]. I tried several times to repeat the findings without success. I also spoke with several colleagues who similarly could not reproduce the work, but none of us ever published our findings. Why not? First off, it is expensive and time consuming to put a paper together for publication, so resources are almost always better spent on other things. Secondly, journals are notorious for not publishing so-called negative results (more on that below). So even though it might be helpful for other scientists to know when a finding is *not* true, one must fight harder with a journal to get these types of papers published. Finally, refuting someone else's work is a good way to make an enemy, and in a world of anonymous peer review, you never know who the person that reviews your next paper or grant will be.

Journals— I have already discussed how a scientific journal's primary incentive is to publish papers that will receive a lot of citations in the first two years after publication, because that is how the <u>Impact Factor</u> is calculated. On the opposite side, there are no consequences to journals for publishing results that are not reproducible. They can simply state that the paper passed peer-review and absolve themselves of any blame, even if their Editors carefully guided a scientist in putting together the experiments for the paper. Furthermore, journals are notoriously reluctant to publish new papers that refute papers they published earlier. Beyond the obvious embarrassment of acknowledging that they published a paper that could not be reproduced, negative-results papers do not get as many citations as other papers, which drags down a journal's Impact Factor.

A good example of this conflict comes from a paper originally published in 2012 in Nature, entitled "Wild-type microglia arrest pathology in a mouse model of Rett syndrome[22]". The original paper made the extraordinary claim that mice genetically altered to have a rare form of autism called Rett syndrome could be treated with bone marrow transplant. Based on these results, the Rett Syndrome Research Trust even began exploring the possibility of performing bone marrow transplants on children with Rett syndrome[23], but to their credit, provided funding to other researchers to replicate the results before proceeding with a clinical trial in humans. So, what happened when four separate scientific teams could not replicate the original findings? Did Nature quickly publish the negative results so that other researchers and families could have access to this information? No, they did not. They extended out the review process before eventually publishing a smaller Brief Communications Arising[24] in 2015 (the original finding was published as a Letter which is featured more prominently in the journal by Nature).

One might be tempted to suggest that this case proves that the system works. Afterall, an organization funded more research to confirm a result before moving on to human trials and the paper contradicting the initial results was published. However, I would argue that it is the exception that proves the rule. The paper was only published because it had the unique situation that four separate labs were willing to come together to publish their results. Even then, the editors at Nature allowed the author of the original article to review the second paper and request experiments to be done before it was accepted for publication. Nature also allowed the original author to write a rebuttal of the second paper. Nature essentially placed their own reputation and the reputation of the original author ahead of the interests of patients, families, funding agencies, and other researchers. In the end, the authors of the original (and likely incorrect) paper still have more citations than the four principal authors of the second paper. As of November 2022, the original paper has 434 citations, while the second paper has 122 citations.

Grant Organizations— Simply put, organizations don't give money to research things that don't work. You can't write a new grant to follow-up on research showing that you cannot reproduce a colleague's work, as it is essentially a dead-end. Unless you are trying to save kids from getting unnecessary bone marrow transplants, you are almost always better served by using that time and money to do your own research than to publish a paper that contradicts another researcher and shows that a certain line of research should not be followed.

The Reproducibility Crisis

In an environment in which the splashiest, most controversial findings are rewarded and there are almost no consequences for publishing incorrect findings, science has become a gigantic hype machine. In my eight years of doing research, I estimate that I was able to replicate about half of published results I tried to reproduce in my own laboratory, and that estimate might be too generous. The Center for Open Science attempted to replicate 193 experiments from top cancer papers published in the years 2010-2012. In 2021, they reported that they could only replicate 50 experiments, or slightly better than 1 in 4. Moreover, of the experiments that they were able to replicate, they found that the sizes of the effects were 85% lower on average than those reported in the original journal articles [25]. Put differently, if a paper reported that a new treatment killed a certain number of cancer cells in the first paper, when the researchers tried to replicate the findings, they found that it killed 85% fewer cancer cells than originally reported. Similar attempts to reproduce findings in psychology (39/100) and economics (11/16) fared slightly better, but they were still far from reassuring[26].

It remains amazing to me that this figure gets so little attention. Imagine the uproar if we found out that over half of the tax-payer money given to the Department of Defense or Medicare or social welfare programs was wasted. It is even more striking considering the important role that biomedical research plays in developing medical treatments for many people. Take the example of Alzheimer's disease, a horrible disorder that causes a loss of neurons in the brain leading to problems with memory and behavior. Alzheimer's disease is a complicated disorder, and for years researchers have been trying to find the underlying cause for the death of the neurons. One of the top theories is that tiny clumps of misfolded proteins called amyloid plaques build up and become toxic to neurons, ultimately leading to their death. This theory is controversial but had many supporters in part due to research published by a scientist named Sylvain Lesné in 2006 in the journal Nature. Sixteen years later, though, it was found that many of the images used in this article were likely manipulated to better support their desired conclusions[27]. Furthermore, a review of other journal articles found that dozens of images in other papers were likely altered as well. In all, manipulated data likely led to tens of millions of dollars of wasted research funding (and time). Worse yet, medications were developed based on the amyloid plaque theory of Alzheimer's disease, potentially exposing patients to risk of medications with little hope of benefit.

The Reality of Academic Research

I want to be clear that I cannot speak for all fields of science. There are likely several fields that produce rigorous, reproducible science. Even in my own field, I am still sometimes amazed at the breakthroughs some scientists can achieve, either through their brilliance or sheer force of will. But the sad reality is that in most cases, the scientific papers themselves, and not the knowledge contained within them, have become the product.

In theory, academic biomedical research is supposed to work in the following way: Money for research comes from either the government or philanthropy (patient advocacy groups or wealthy donors) to fund basic and translational research. Scientists publish their findings in journals to expand the body of new knowledge with the hope that it will advance the field and lead to new ways to diagnose, prevent, or treat diseases.

In practice, academic research has mostly become an echo chamber, completely isolated from either the clinical practice of medicine or the efforts of biomedical companies to produce new treatments. Publishing in prestigious journals and generating headlines in news releases has replaced actual scientific knowledge, because research is now mostly funded by the two most unpopular groups in the United States: the federal government and the ultra-wealthy who use the illusion of progress as a way of white washing their reputation. It is much easier to highlight the opening of a hospital wing, or endowing a Professorship, or the provision of funding to research a disease than it is to make actual progress. Until the groups that fund research compel the scientific establishment to produce rigorous, reproducible findings, then the current situation is unlikely to change.

Chapter 4: Evidence-Based Medicine

In recent years, the concept of evidence-based medicine has swept through medicine. The basic premise of evidence-based medicine is that when there are multiple treatments available for a condition, these treatments should be compared head-to-head in research studies to identify the safest and most effective treatments. Medical providers can then use this information along with their clinical judgment and the patient's preferences to make the best possible treatment decisions. In Chapter 4, I will outline the principles of evidence-based medicine and discuss how in real practice, profits are what drive medical decision making.

Evidence-based medicine (or evidence-based practice for fields like psychology and nutrition) refers to a movement that began in the 1990s to integrate empirical data from large research studies into patient care. Prior to this, much of the medical care provided by doctors was based largely upon either what they learned from the doctors that they trained with in medical school and residency or from their own personal experience. This arrangement may have worked well enough for less severe conditions, but it caused serious concerns for diseases like cancer where patient outcomes could vary widely between treatment centers.

The key component of evidence-based medicine is the randomized-controlled trial. Randomized-controlled trials are conducted by taking large groups of patients with the same or similar illnesses and dividing them into two or more groups at random. This random assignment is critical to make sure that the groups are truly equal. For example, imagine a study that compared a new cancer treatment to the current standard treatment. If patients were allowed to pick which treatment they received, then patients who are sicker or who have failed to get better from standard treatments may be more likely to choose the new treatment out of desperation. It is hard to compare two treatments if the patients in each group are not relatively equal. Imagine in the example above where a cancer patient in a research study is allowed to pick the treatment that they receive. If patients who got the new treatment had worse results, it could be because the new treatment really was worse *or* it could be because only the patients who were sicker chose to receive the new treatment, so they were less likely to get better to begin with. Without ensuring that the two groups are balanced, it's impossible to know if a treatment works or not.

The second important part of a randomized controlled trial is the control group, which is used to compare the treatment group to. Not only are patients not allowed to choose their group, but they are also not told which group they will be placed into until the trial has ended. This is called a blinded study because the patient is 'blind' to the group that they have been placed in. Blinding is important because knowing which group they are in may affect a patient's outcome. While knowing if you receive a medication or placebo may not affect things like blood pressure or cholesterol level, it could affect how a patient reports their anxiety, for instance, in a study of anxiety medication. A study is said to be double-blinded if neither the patient in the study nor the person conducting the study knows which group the patient is assigned to. This double blinding is important to eliminate any bias on the part of the researcher who might be tempted to skew results if they knew which patient was receiving which treatment.

The standard control group in a medication study is a <u>placebo</u> (which is sometimes called a sugar pill), but essentially is just the treatment with no medication included in it. Control groups can be more difficult to design when the treatment is not a medication. For instance, think of research studies that look at things like the effects of psychotherapy, exercise, or a change in your diet. There is no easy way to give a placebo for an exercise routine or change in your diet without the patient knowing (so the study is no longer 'blinded'). One option is to use a <u>waitlist control group</u>. In this situation, some of the patients that volunteer for the study are put into a 'wait list' group that does not receive treatment until later. For the purpose of the research study, individuals on the waitlist are then compared to the patients who did receive the treatment, but those patients on the waitlist eventually receive treatment themselves after the study has concluded[28]. One important thing to remember is that waitlist trials are usually not blinded. It is obvious to tell, for instance, if someone received the treatment or not.

Placebo pills and waitlist control groups are fine when there are no good treatments available or when there are minimal long-term consequences of not getting treatment for an illness (like having the patient's cholesterol be too high for a few months). It becomes a more complicated ethical question when there is a known treatment for a condition and withholding it might cause long-term harm. For instance, in the field of psychiatry, the Food and Drug Administration requires that patients must be taken off their medications before a clinical trial and then randomly assigned into the treatment or control group (which is usually a placebo). Therefore, most of the information that we get from clinical trials submitted to the Food and Drug Administration only show if a treatment is **better than nothing.** Again, this is fine if there are no other treatments available but is not terribly helpful when there are multiple treatments already available (which are usually less expensive and have a longer history of safety data).

Therefore, most of the studies that make up the basis of evidence-based medicine come from trials funded by the government or non-profit organizations. These studies can be broadly divided into two groups: <u>efficacy</u> studies vs. <u>effectiveness</u> studies. In both types of research, a treatment is being compared to a control (this again is mostly placebo but may be a standard treatment that is already available). The major difference between the two types of studies is the conditions under which they are done. An efficacy study is typically conducted under 'ideal conditions' in which you would be most likely to see a difference. Ideal conditions can involve many different things, but they almost always involve limiting who is allowed to participate in the study. For instance, in psychiatry, a researcher may want to test a new medication for patients with binge eating disorder to see if it reduces episodes of binge eating. In this case, the researcher may choose to eliminate anyone with a history of drug addiction, depression, anxiety, psychosis, or a serious medical problem from participating in the study because all those conditions would make it less likely that the medication would work or more likely that a patient would have a side effect to the medication.

Efficacy studies also carefully select other things that might influence the likelihood that a treatment will work, such as where the research is done or who conducts it. Many research studies are conducted at medical schools and universities with highly trained staff. This can be especially important for treatments like psychotherapy, for which the skill of the therapist is important to the overall outcome of the treatment. Efficacy studies are often done for new treatments to see if they work at all. Research studies are very expensive and take a long time, so it makes sense to do a small study first under ideal conditions to see if the treatment works at all before moving on to larger, more costly studies. The major drawback of an efficacy study is that it may not be relevant to most patients with an illness who don't have access to treatment under ideal conditions.

Unlike efficacy studies, effectiveness research focuses more on 'real world conditions.' An effectiveness study will have fewer reasons to reject a patient who wants to participate and will usually be conducted by research staff that is more typically found in the community. These studies tend to be more helpful in treating patients outside of research settings, but are also much larger, more expensive, and harder to conduct. Therefore, fewer of them have been done. In the late 1990s and early 2000s, the National Institute of Mental Health conducted three large effectiveness studies for major depression, bipolar disorder, and schizophrenia. The results were bleak. I already reported the findings for the study on major depression (STAR*D), which found that a third of patients had not recovered after 4 medications. The bipolar disorder study (STEP-BD) achieved recovery for 58% of patients by the end of the study, but almost one half of recovered patients later had their symptoms return[29]. The schizophrenia study (CATIE) tried to compare different antipsychotic medications to see which ones were most effective at reducing symptoms of psychosis, but this question could not be answered because almost three-quarters of patients (74%) stopped taking their medications within the 18 months of the study[30].

<u>Best Practices</u>

Once there have been a series of studies on the treatment of a specific disease like diabetes, epilepsy, or rheumatoid arthritis, experts (usually professional organizations) will get together, review all the research findings, and put together a list of best practices or treatment algorithms that give step-by-step recommendations on how to treat a specific illness. These recommendations are highly influential and sway billions of dollars of healthcare spending. Each recommendation in a best practice guideline will often come with a ranking of the quality of evidence. At the very top of the list are large randomized controlled trials (preferably more than one study) that compare multiple treatments head-to-head. On the low end of the quality scale are things like <u>case reports</u> (in which a single patient or small group of patients has responded to a specific treatment) or <u>expert opinion</u> (which basically consists of the recommendations of famous researchers).

Eventually, once multiple treatments have been studied for long enough, it is possible to come up with something called the <u>number needed to treat</u> (sometimes called the NNT). The number needed to treat is basically a statistic that tells you how many people need to receive a certain treatment to get a specific benefit. The number needed to treat can be a little confusing to understand at first, so it may be helpful to give an example. Let's say for instance that a new medication has been developed to prevent someone from having a stroke. During the time of the study, 2% of people without the treatment have a stroke while 1% of those on the medication have a stroke. That means for every 100 who received treatment, 2 people who did not receive treatment had a stroke, while 1 person who received treatment had a stroke. You can use this information to then calculate the Number Needed to Treat, or number of people you need to treat to prevent a stroke. In this example the answer is 100, that is, 100 patients need to take this medication to prevent one stroke. The same calculation can also be done for side effects to find something called the <u>number needed to harm,</u> or NNH. For instance, if 2% of control patients in the study have a severe episode of bleeding compared to 4% of patients who receive the medication, then the Number Needed to Harm is 50. For every 50 patients who received the medication, 1 additional person will have severe bleeding.

The number needed to treat can be used as a quick method to understand how likely you are to benefit (or be harmed) from a treatment. A group called TheNNT has published a fascinating list showing the number needed to treat (and number needed to harm) for various treatments at TheNNT.com. For instance, in elderly patients living in a nursing home, vitamin D helped prevent hip fractures (NNT of 36) but also increased the rate of kidney stones (NNH of

36). So, if you give vitamin D to a group of nursing home patients, you need to treat 36 patients to prevent one hip fracture, but you will also cause one extra person to have a kidney stone who would not have otherwise had one[31]. Patients and families can then use these numbers to compare the relative risk vs benefit of a potential treatment.

<u>There Is No Evidence-based Practice</u>

In recent years, there has been a major focus on "evidence-based practice." The basic idea is that treatment providers should strive to use the most effective treatments identified by academic researchers (the "evidence") as the basis for the care that they provide. In theory, this sounds nice, and I have found that many treatment programs love to claim that they use "evidence-based practice", but as someone who has seen how research is done and how clinical care is actually delivered, I have found that the majority of the care in psychiatry does not meet the standards of "evidence-based practice."

The first challenge to the idea of evidence-based practice is that the scientific literature is systematically flawed. As I mentioned previously, most major scientific studies cannot be reproduced, so the very "evidence" on which these guidelines are published is suspect. The National Institute of Mental Health has largely abandoned researching new treatments[32], and as a result, the studies that are published are often skewed. For instance, pharmaceutical companies specifically design studies to show their medications in a favorable way, and most studies only compare a medication to placebo, which is of very limited use when you are trying to compare multiple treatment options.

There is also a well-known publication bias in that studies with good results are much more likely to be published and promoted than studies with negative results[33]. Research studies that are done with National Institute of Health funding are usually published in scientific journals that you have to have a subscription to read. In contrast, pharmaceutical companies will pay to have the articles that they publish freely available to the public or medical providers. The result is that most of the clinical information that is easily accessible to medical providers highlights medications that are still under patent (so there is no generic version available) and are thus profitable for pharmaceutical companies to study.

The final major obstacle to evidence-based practice is that in most of the academic programs that train medical providers, therapists, and dietitians, there is very little interaction between the researchers and the clinicians[34]. Because of this separation, I find that most clinicians have very limited knowledge on how research is conducted and therefore what the research actually shows.

Let's take the example of research on a medication used to treat a psychiatric diagnosis like major depression, schizophrenia, or bipolar disorder. First, in a research study, the official diagnosis is made by an interview called the Structured Diagnostic Interview for DSM (often referred to as a 'SCID'). These interviews are considered 'scripted' because it literally lays out step by step the exact questions to ask about each sign and symptom of a mental illness. Depending on the answers to the questions, the script then tells the interviewer to either ask more questions or skip to the next section. This continues repeatedly until almost 300 diagnoses are covered. These interviews can take anywhere from an hour to several hours depending on a person's history. At the end, a very specific diagnosis is reached that is supposed to be very consistent no matter who is doing the interview. I don't know anyone in clinical practice who uses the Structured Clinical Interview for DSM to diagnose patients. In fact, I once suggested to the Director of our psychiatry residency program that psychiatry residents should observe a Structured Clinical Interview for DSM *once* in their training so that they can understand who gets included or excluded from a clinical trial, and I was told unequivocally that not only would this not be useful, but that it would be counterproductive to the practice of psychiatry. So, from the very start, there is a huge difference between the carefully selected patients who get to participate in the research studies and the patients who are treated on a day-to-day basis.

Once a patient is formally given a diagnosis, they then enter a research trial in which the medication and dose prescribed is based upon predetermined criteria using questionnaires to measure someone's symptoms. For instance, consider a trial on major depression. The study may only enroll patients with a score of moderate to severe symptoms of depression on the survey questionnaire. A patient would be given the starting dose of a medication and then come back several weeks later and take the survey questionnaire again, and the decision to adjust the dose of the medication would be based upon how they score on the survey questionnaire. If the patient still scores in the moderate to severe range, then the medication dose would be increased. If the patient's depression symptoms are now either gone or mild, then the dose may stay the same. The patient will continue to return for visits and retake the survey questionnaire with the dose of the medication being adjusted up or down based upon their responses.

I cannot speak on all the outpatient treatment in the world, and I am sure that there are some very well-trained clinicians who provide excellent care, but for the vast majority of Inpatient or Residential treatment programs that I am familiar with, the current state of psychiatric treatment more closely resembles "profit-based medicine" than "evidence-based medicine." Medical providers like psychiatrists or nurse practitioners see patients for a few minutes a week. Many times, self-report questionnaires have replaced a diagnostic interview to diagnose patients in order to save time (something that self-report questionnaires were never designed to do).

The examples that I gave above are for the prescription of a medication, but there are similar problems with the psychotherapy that is delivered as well. Studies that test new psychotherapies must be <u>manualized</u> so that each therapy session is written out step by step. The therapists delivering the care in research studies must also be videotaped and scored to make sure they are correctly delivering the psychotherapy. Most of the psychotherapy provided in treatment centers is done either by interns getting in clinical hours in order to get their full license or by new therapists fresh out of school, because these are the least expensive people to hire. Likewise, much of the therapy that is performed is done in a group setting because it is much more cost effective to have 10 patients sit through a 1-hour group than to do 10 hours of individual psychotherapy. I am not aware of any treatment programs where therapists use treatment manuals or record sessions to grade the quality of care that the therapists are providing.

The best analogy that I have for the gap between the treatments that appear in research journals and the actual care that is delivered to patients is a restaurant. University researchers are like celebrity chefs. They work under ideal conditions, have the most talented assistants, and large amounts of time and money to develop new products, which they can go around the country promoting. Treatment centers, on the other hand, are like a chain of fast-food restaurants. Their job is to take something developed under ideal conditions and find a way to mass produce it in a way that makes the maximum profit. In the end, their work may resemble the original, but will never meet the same quality level.

Chapter 5: Modern Psychiatry's Original Sin

In this chapter, I will lay out the background on how psychiatric disorders are diagnosed, how the causes of these disorders and their potential treatments are researched and provide background information about genetics and how genetic mutations increase the risk of developing a psychiatric disorder. This information will lead us to an understanding of the faults in our current approach to psychiatric treatment and the need for precision psychiatry.

The Diagnostic and Statistical Manual-III created a common language to describe the <u>signs</u> and <u>symptoms</u> of mental illness and grouped those signs and symptoms into a series of disorders or syndromes. One initial goal of this change in the Diagnostic and Statistical Manual-III was to improve communication between treatment providers. Terms like manic depression, bipolar disorder, and cyclic insanity were used interchangeably by different clinicians throughout the world[35]. By standardizing a set of criteria for each diagnosis and making each criterion more objectively defined, it made it easier for treatment providers to understand what issues a patient was dealing with.

This approach had another, broader consequence though. Because signs and symptoms of a mental illness can be reported or observed, they have the advantage of also being measurable. So how do you measure something like sadness? The answer is by creating questionnaires or surveys that have patients rate their symptoms. Take for example a question from the Quick Inventory of Depressive Symptoms-Self Report (QIDS-SR)[36]:

Check the one response to each item that best represents you for the past seven days....

Feeling sad:

- I do not feel sad.

- I feel sad less than half the time.

- I feel sad more than half the time.

- I feel sad nearly all of the time.

The Quick Inventory of Depressive Symptoms-Self Report questionnaire asks the person to answer several questions like this for different symptoms of major depressive disorder each with four answers, including the example above, about feeling sad. Each answer is worth between 0 and 3 points depending how severe your symptoms are for each of the depression criteria. In the example above, the first answer "I do not feel sad" would be worth 0 points while the last answer "I feel sad nearly all of the time" would be worth 3 points. Once a patient gets through all the questions in the survey, the points can be added up to get a depression score between 0 and 27, with 0 to 5 being 'no depression', 6 to 10 being 'mild depression', 11 to 15 'moderate depression', 16 to 20 'severe depression', and over 21 as 'very severe depression'. The Quick Inventory of Depressive Symptoms-Self Report survey is for major depression, but similar questions can be asked to come up with a survey to measure the symptoms of many disorders, including bipolar disorder, obsessive-compulsive disorders, and substance abuse.

Once a disorder can be consistently diagnosed and measured, it opens a wide variety of questions that can be asked. For instance, researchers can measure how many people have a diagnosis in a particular time frame. This is called the prevalence of a disorder and can help public health officials determine how much treatment needs to be available for a specific condition. A researcher may want to measure how many new cases of a disorder will be diagnosed in a year. This is called the incidence of a disorder and indicates if a disease is increasing or decreasing in the population. A researcher might also want to measure the age at which a patient is most likely to get a new diagnosis of a disorder. This measure is called peak incidence. For example, if the peak incidence of binge drinking is 23 years old, it means that 23 is the most common age for people to begin binge drinking. Knowing the peak incidence of a disease can be used to help screen for an illness or in efforts to prevent it, such as focusing efforts to prevent binge drinking on the 18-23 age group in the example above.

The next logical step is to use the symptom score from a questionnaire to measure how well a treatment works or does not work for a specific diagnosis. Let's say that a patient has a score of 20 on their depression scale (severe), you can now see if a specific treatment like a medication reduces that score. If a patient diagnosed with major depression receives treatment and their score drops to the 0 to 5 range, then they are said to be recovered because they no longer have symptoms of depression. If their score drops by at least 50% but remains above 5 (the cut off to be considered mildly depressed) then they are said to have responded. In the example above, a treatment could reduce the score from 20 to 9. In this case, the patient would still be classified as mildly depressed, but they have *responded* to the treatment because they have fewer symptoms.

How Psychiatry Became Paralyzed

There is nothing wrong with any of these initial studies using Diagnostic and Statistical Manual criteria. All of them, to some extent, provided information that was helpful for the diagnosis, treatment, or prevention of certain illnesses. What is more difficult to explain is how this decision sent psychiatry down a specific path that is now difficult to change. The university research system is highly hierarchical.

Individual professors spend years studying a specific disease or treatment and build their reputations through publishing a series of papers on that topic. In turn, they train the next generation of researchers who build their own careers by following up on these findings. Once a researcher gets to the top of their field, they become highly invested in maintaining their status, which means not having their work challenged. Not only do top researchers have a strong incentive not to see their work refuted, but they also have significant leverage to make sure that does not happen. In the hierarchical system, the top researchers typically are the ones reviewing grants, papers, and nominees for awards or prizes. They organize the conferences that people attend and decide who is going to speak at them. They are typically involved in the process of hiring new faculty and deciding upon promotion. Challenging the work of a top researcher in your field can be professional suicide.

The result of this is that academic research is not adept at changing direction. While researchers at a pharmaceutical company may shut down an entire research program if they are not making progress toward a drug that can get Food and Drug Administration approval, there is no equivalent in academic research. Professors who are highly invested in maintaining the *status quo* continue to push their ideas long after it has been useful. Put differently, if someone has built their career studying major depressive disorder or bipolar disorder or schizophrenia, then there is a strong incentive not to see those disorders go away and erase a lifetime of work.

This is essentially what the National Institute of Mental Health tried to do several years ago. The National Institute of Mental Health was rightly criticized for the lack of new treatments for psychiatric diagnoses coming from the research that they had funded. Almost all the medications currently used to treat mental illness were discovered by accident decades before. Despite all the money that has been poured into research over the years, scientists have not rationally designed a treatment for major depression, bipolar disorder, schizophrenia, autism spectrum disorder, anxiety, obsessive compulsive disorder, or eating disorders. The scientists at the National Institute of Mental Health felt that the major reason why the research they funded failed to find new treatments for psychiatric disorders was because the diagnostic criteria set forth by the Diagnostic and Statistical Manual lacked validity and was not an accurate reflection of what was causing mental illness in the brain[37]. That is, the makers of the Diagnostic and Statistical Manual 'lumped' together illnesses that had similar symptoms (like feeling sad or experiencing psychosis) even though those illnesses had different underlying causes.

The National Institute of Mental Health decided that it needed to spend years developing their own framework for classifying mental illness to replace the Diagnostic and Statistical Manual, called the Research Domain Criteria. The Research Domain Criteria identified five distinct areas of brain functioning that could be affected in mental illness[38]. The goal may have been to make it easier for neuroscientists to do research, but unfortunately, no one else was bound by it. The authors of the Diagnostic and Statistical Manual had no incentive to discard years of research that they built their careers on, and the American Psychiatric Association was not going to give up a major source of income like publishing the Diagnostic and Statistical Manual. Pharmaceutical companies were only accountable to the Food and Drug Administration to approve their products and not the National Institute of Mental Health. The Food and Drug Administration had no incentive to buck the American Psychiatric Association and pharmaceutical industry to support researchers funded by the National Institute of Mental Health. As of now, the fate of the Research Domain Criteria system as an alternative to traditional Diagnostic and

Statistical Manual criteria remains in limbo[39], but serves as a stark warning to those who attempt to change the *status quo*.

So why don't pharmaceutical companies attempt to buck the current Diagnostic and Statistical Manual system? I have far less interaction with the pharmaceutical industry, but from talking to colleagues who have worked at pharmaceutical companies, my impression is that they have financial incentives to maintain the current system. Broadly speaking, psychiatric medications only fall within a few small categories. The first class of medications increase levels of monoamine neurotransmitters like serotonin, dopamine, and norepinephrine. This group of medications are often called 'antidepressants' because of their prevalent use to treat major depression, but medications from this group are also used to treat a broad range of diagnoses, including generalized anxiety disorder, panic disorder, obsessive compulsive disorder, social anxiety, post-traumatic stress disorder, premenstrual dysphoric disorder, and bulimia nervosa. The second major group of medication generally work by blocking the dopamine-2 receptor (there are five dopamine receptors in total) and are often referred to as the antipsychotics because of their frequent use to treat psychosis in schizophrenia and schizoaffective disorder, but they are also used widely to treat bipolar disorder, treatment resistant major depression, and autism spectrum disorder. The third class are the stimulant medications like methylphenidate and dextroamphetamine/ amphetamine, and they work by increasing the release of dopamine from neurons in the brain and are used primarily to treat attention deficit hyperactivity disorder (ADHD), but are also used for binge eating disorder, narcolepsy, and treatment resistant depression (especially in the elderly). The fourth group are sedative medications that increase the action of the inhibitory neurotransmitter GABA and include benzodiazepines (like Xanax) and certain sleep medications (including Ambien). Sedatives are used for panic attacks, insomnia, generalized anxiety disorder, specific phobia, and to treat alcohol withdrawal symptoms. The final class is lithium, an electrolyte like sodium or potassium, but with psychoactive properties. Lithium is most recognized for treatment of mania in bipolar disorder, but is also used for treatment resistant depression, especially when there is strong suicidal ideation.

These five classes of medication, all originally discovered incidentally in the 1950s and 1960s, account for most of the treatment in psychiatry. While we know the neurotransmitters that these medications target in the brain, for the most part, we still don't know *how* they work. The fact that these five classes of medications can be used to treat such a broad range of diagnoses suggests that they have general benefits to neuron function far removed from the actual cause of the illness. Anti-inflammatory medications like corticosterone and ibuprofen are a good comparison for this idea. Both corticosterone and ibuprofen are used to decrease pain and inflammation for a broad range of conditions, but neither one treats the underlying cause of the pain or inflammation. In the same way, psychiatric medications help relieve the symptoms of many conditions, but don't treat the actual underlying cause, which explains why they *help a little bit for a lot of conditions.*

My theory is that it is more profitable for pharmaceutical companies to continue to make slightly updated versions of these five medication classes with a wide market than it is to find a new treatment for a smaller subset of patients. This creates a conflict between the financial incentives of pharmaceutical companies, who benefit from marketing drugs that *help a little bit for a lot of things,* and patients, who would prefer treatments that *help a lot for their specific condition.* You can see this tension play out in other areas of medicine like gene therapy. There are now treatments for very rare genetic disorders, but because the number of patients affected is so low, the cost of the treatment must be hundreds of thousands of dollars each to cover the cost of developing the treatment[40], which greatly limits access to these treatments. Until the financial benefits of broadly inclusive diagnostic criteria are addressed, I am worried that we will not see new approaches to treating psychiatric illness.

<u>Current Methods to Study Psychiatric Illness</u>

Psychiatry has always been hampered in ways that other fields of medicine have not. The human brain is quite different even from its closest ancestors, the chimpanzees, while other organs like the heart, liver, and kidneys are broadly similar, even down to lab animals like rats and mice. The central nervous system is also encased in a thick layer of bone, which makes getting tissue samples very difficult. The closest comparison would be the field of neurology, which is also interested in dysfunction of the brain. Neurology, though, has the advantage of studying several diseases in which you can either observe physical changes in the brain by CT scan or MRI (like stroke or multiple sclerosis), or that cause dramatic change in brain wave activity that can be picked up by monitors (like seizures).

The field of psychiatry remained largely descriptive until the 1980s and 1990s when new technologies became available to study the brains of awake human beings. Brain imaging studies like <u>SPECT</u> (Single-photon emission computed tomography) and <u>functional MRI</u> (also referred to as fMRI) allowed researchers to look at the activity of different brain regions for the first time. SPECT scans use a radioactive material injected into the body to measure blood flow in the brain. Functional MRI works in a slightly different way. Whereas a traditional MRI just shows a 3-D picture of the brain, functional MRI can measure when a part of the brain becomes active. Functional MRI can do this because when a brain region becomes active it uses more oxygen, so the amount of oxygen bound to the hemoglobin in the red blood cells drops slightly. Importantly, there is a difference in the magnetic properties of hemoglobin with and without oxygen, and this difference can be detected by an MRI machine. So, in functional MRI, a researcher can determine if a brain region becomes more or less active by measuring small changes in the amount of oxygen consumed in that brain region.

One key feature of functional MRI, though, is that it requires a 'task'. That is, the person must be doing something in the MRI machine like looking at a picture or playing a game. The researcher then measures the activity of the brain at rest and then compares it to the brain activity while performing the task to detect a difference. This is what makes an MRI 'functional', it looks at a brain that is engaged in an activity. There is a wide range of tasks that can be performed during a functional MRI scan, including looking at specific images, playing games, and tasting a specific food. For example, a researcher may look at the brain activity of a person with bipolar disorder playing a game that involves gambling to see if there is a region of the brain that regulates risk taking behaviors.

These approaches can give great insight into how changes in the activity of certain brain regions can produce symptoms of mental illness. However, there are a few limitations to brain imaging studies. First, the task must be relevant to the disorder being studied. Moreover, the task must be able to be performed by a person within an MRI machine. These machines are very large cylinders with just enough space for a human to fit inside, they have loud spinning magnets in the cylinder, and a person must remain laying down and their head must remain very still during the experiment, all of which obviously limit what tasks can be done during an experiment. Moreover, functional imaging scans are not powerful enough to draw conclusions for an individual person because the effect is so small and difficult to measure. Instead, brain scans on large groups of people with an illness vs. people in a control group (that is, a group of people without the illness) must be combined into a dataset and compared. So, while functional MRI can be useful to investigate brain regions involved in a particular disease or behavior, it is not helpful for the diagnosis or treatment of an individual.

<u>Background on Genetics</u>

Genetic studies are another area that promised to revolutionize the understanding of mental illness. The risk of developing a mental illness is partly inherited from your parents and partly due to the environment during development. The inherited risk is derived mostly from the DNA each parent contributes at conception.

DNA is like a recipe book describing how to make the more than 20,000 different proteins your body needs to function. DNA is composed of 4 separate letters (A, T, C, G) that form one long continuous sentence that is 6 billion letters long. Instead of spelling words, however, the A, T, C and Gs of DNA spell out amino acids by forming three letter combinations called codons. For instance, the three-letter combination ATG in DNA is the instruction for the amino acid methionine.

<u>Amino acids</u> are molecules composed of a carbon atom at the center that has four other atoms or combinations of atoms attached to it. There is a nitrogen atom with three hydrogens (the amino part), a carbon atom with two oxygens (the acid part), a hydrogen atom, and a variable side chain. The side chain is an additional combination of atoms that makes each individual amino acid unique. Some side chains are small, some side chains are positively charged or negatively charged like the side of a magnet, some are large and avoid water like an oil, some have special atoms in them like sulfur that can undergo unique chemical reactions. Overall, there are 20 amino acids that are used to make proteins in the human body. Importantly, the body can only make 11 out of the 20 amino acids, which means that the remaining nine amino acids are 'essential' to have in your diet (see illustration on next page).

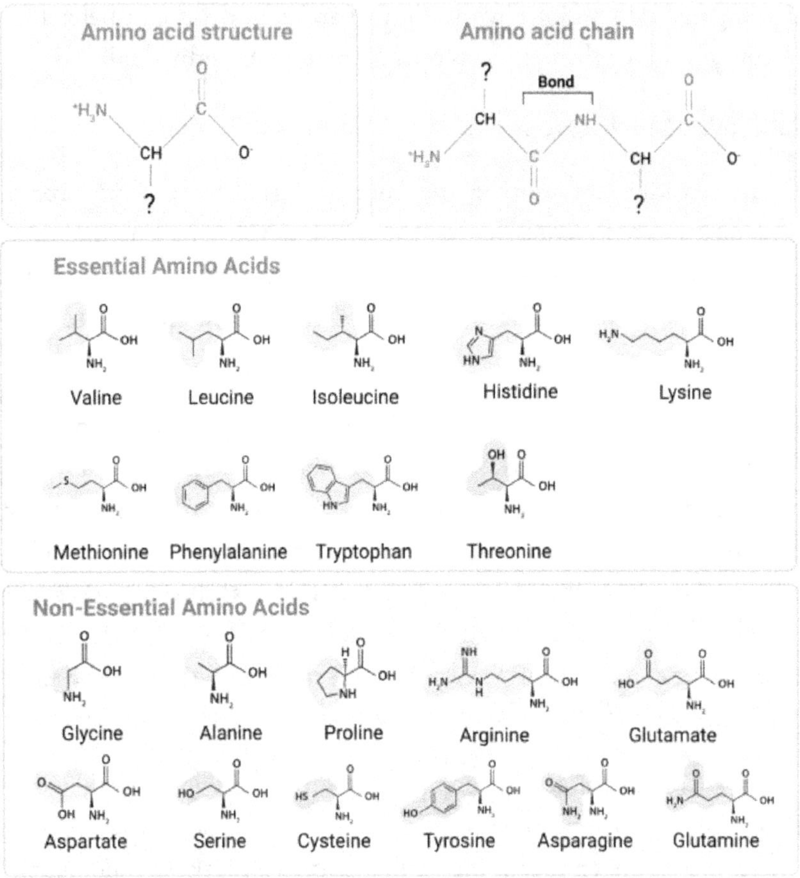

Essential Amino Acids

Non-Essential Amino Acids

Amino Acids: the upper left box shows the structure of an amino acid. Each amino acid is composed of a carbon molecule with four thing attached to: nitrogen atom with three hydrogen atoms (the amino part), a carbon atom with two oxygen atoms (the acid part), a hydrogen atom, and a variable side chain (shown as a '?'). The upper right box shows how the 'amino' end of one amino acid can form a bond with the 'acid' end of another amino to link the two together in a chain. There are twenty different side chains that can appear in amino acids, each with different chemical properties. The middle box shows nine amino acids that the body can not make on its own so they are 'essential' to have in the foods that you eat. The bottom box shows the remaining 11 non-essential amino acids.

When a protein is made, the 'amino' end and the 'acid' end are linked together like two train cars to form a chain. The A, T, C, and G of DNA can create 64 different 3-letter combinations. 61 of those combinations correspond to one of the 20 amino acids while the remaining 3 combinations are 'stop' codons that tell the cell to stop making the protein. A gene gives instructions to the cell in the specific order that each amino acid must be put in place to form a particular protein (see illustration on next page).

It is the combination of how these 20 different amino acids are strung together that creates the incredible variety of proteins in your body. Proteins may initially start off as a thin line of amino acids like a row of train cars or the beads on a necklace, but as soon as they are made, they begin to fold into different shapes based upon the order of the amino acids and how they interact with each other and the other contents of the cell. Small proteins can be a few hundred amino acids long, while a larger protein can go into the thousands, so the variety of shapes and functions that proteins can take is astonishing. Even a small protein that is only 200 amino acids long, in theory, could have over 10,000,000,000,000,000,000,000,000,000 different combinations of the 20 amino acids!

You have likely heard of many of the proteins found in the body. For instance, collagen is a structural protein that gives strength to connective tissues like tendons and skin. Proteins in your muscle called actin and myosin interact causing muscle fibers to contract which allows your body to move. Digestive enzymes break down the food that you eat, like lipases (for breaking down fats), proteinases (for proteins), and amylases (for starch). Antibodies are proteins produced by your immune system that can bind to bacteria or viruses that infect the body. Hemoglobin is the protein in your red blood cells which carries oxygen from your lungs to the rest of your body through the blood vessels. There are over 20,000 different genes that give instructions on how to make proteins in the body (plus more variation if you include the ability of the cell to use different parts of a gene to make slightly different versions of the protein, called a splice variant).

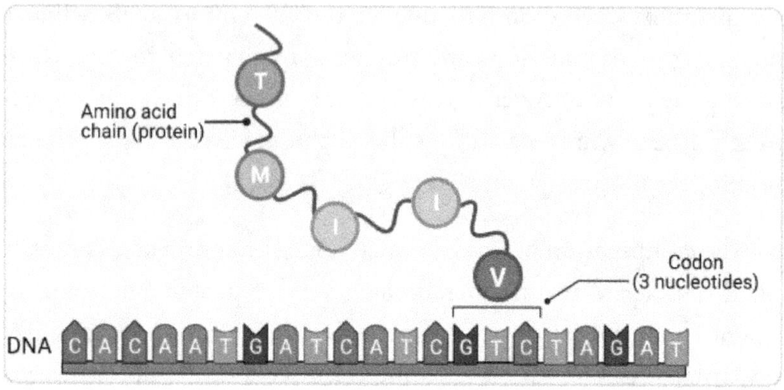

How DNA codes for proteins: DNA molecules contain a string of 4 letters- A, C, T, and G. Groups of 3 letters are called a 'codon'. Each 3-letter codon represents a different amino acid. In the example above, the 3-letter combination GTG tells the cell to add the amino acid valine next in line to the growing protein.

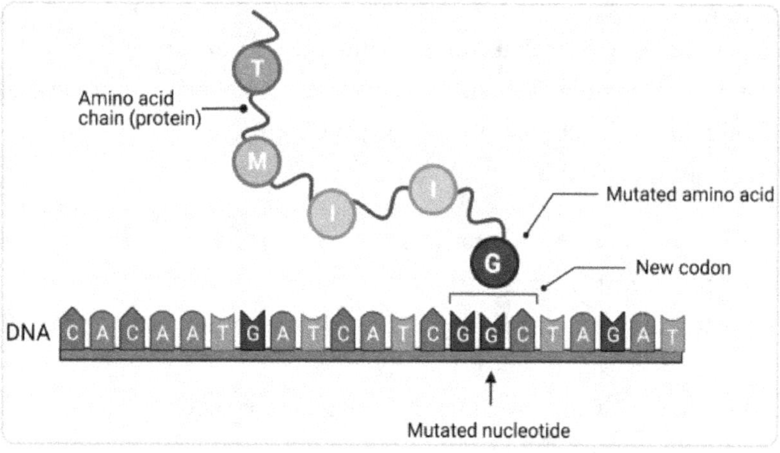

How genetic mutations change proteins: Mutations occur when there is a change to the letters in the DNA. In the example above the 'T' is changed to a 'G' which changes the codon from GTC to GGC. The new GGC codon now tells the cell to place the amino acid glycine in the protein chain instead of valine.

Each person has two copies of almost every gene that they get from each parent[41]. It is like inheriting a full set of cookbooks with over 20,000 recipes from each parent. Sometimes there are changes made in these recipes when your DNA is copied. Imagine writing down one of your parent's recipes by hand and accidentally changing the 'Tsp' to 'Tbsp' for the amount of salt to add. The next time you make the recipe you might accidentally put in a Tbsp (tablespoon) of salt instead of a Tsp (teaspoon). From then on, every time someone else copied the recipe down, their recipe would also have the incorrect directions for the amount of salt as well.

Whenever there is a change in the letters of DNA it is called a genetic variant. In this book, I will distinguish between a genetic variant and a genetic mutation, because many changes in DNA have little to no consequences. I will use the term genetic variant to describe a change in the DNA that is not known to have any consequences on biological functioning, and genetic mutation to refer to a change in the DNA sequence that causes a change in functioning (mutations can be helpful or damaging). In the example above, the slight increase in salt may not change the taste of the recipe very much at all, so you could consider this to be a *variation* in the recipe. Now, let's say that for the same recipe you accidentally copy down '113' cups instead of '⅓' cups for the chili powder. This change would significantly alter the taste of a recipe, which you could call a *mutation* in the recipe.

Sickle cell anemia is an example of a disease that is caused by a genetic mutation. In sickle cell anemia, there is a mutation in the gene that provides the directions for making hemoglobin— the protein that carries oxygen in your blood cells. If you inherit one bad copy of the gene from one parent, you have sickle trait. Individuals with sickle trait have a less severe form of the illness and often do not have symptoms unless they get into certain situations, like the low oxygen level environment that occurs at high altitude. If you receive two bad copies of the hemoglobin gene, then you have sickle cell anemia, in which case the hemoglobin sticks together in clumps, changing the red blood cell from a round, donut shape to the characteristic sickle shape that gives the disease its name.

Genetic Research

Genetic research is especially attractive to researchers studying mental illness. As mentioned before, researchers have a hard time getting samples of human brain tissues, and lab animals like mice are of limited use for many phenomena important to psychiatric research, like hallucinations and suicide. DNA, on the other hand, is quite easy to obtain from a cheek cell swab or blood draw. Genetic risk is also very important to the risk of developing a psychiatric diagnosis from autism and schizophrenia, for which the risk is mostly inherited, to major depression and post-traumatic stress disorder, for which environmental factors like abuse, neglect, or stress take a larger role in the likelihood of developing the illness.

Mental illness is considered polygenic, which basically means that mutations affecting many different genes can all contribute to the risk, as opposed to a monogenic illness like sickle cell anemia in which there is a single gene causing the disease. While we know that thousands of different genetic changes can increase the risk of developing an illness, not all mutations increase this risk the same amount. Genetic variants vary largely in both how common they are in the population and in how much they increase the risk of developing an illness (see illustration on next page).

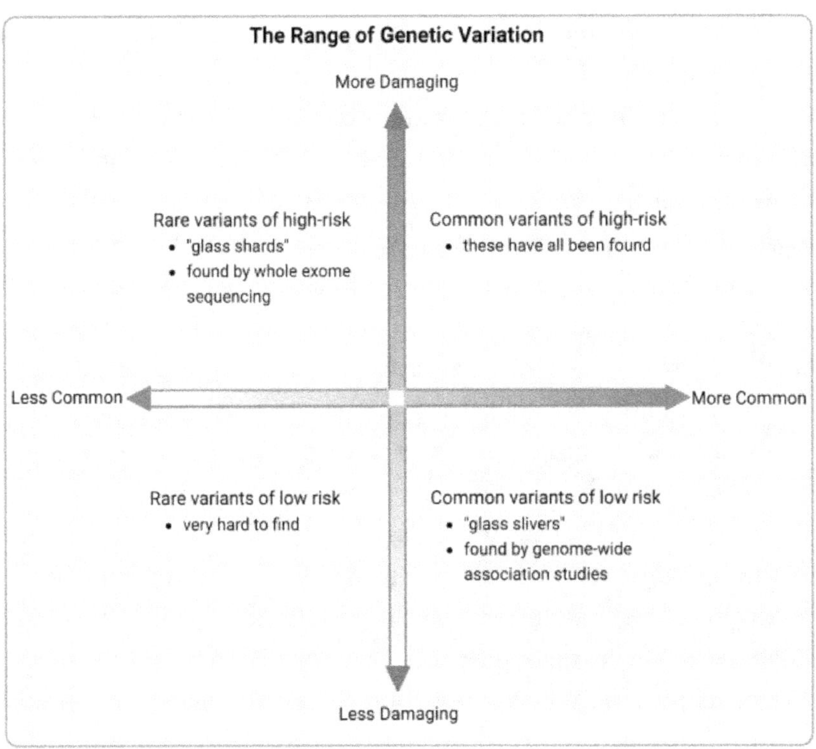

The Range of Genetic Variation: You can broadly think of risk causing mutations in four different groups depending on how common they are in the population (blue line) and how damaging they are to the protein they make (red line). The first group of genetic mutations are common and significantly increase your risk of having an illness like sickle cell disease where 1 in 13 people of black or African American descent are born with one copy of the genetic mutation that causes sickle cell disease (upper right). The second group are genetic mutations which are very common in the population (>1% usually), but each mutation increases your risk of getting an illness by only a small amount (lower right). The third group consists of variants that are rare, like 1 in 100,000, 1 in a million, or never seen before, but greatly increase your chance of having an illness (upper left). The so-called breast cancer genes *BRCA1* and *BRCA2* are good examples of these types of variants. Mutations in *BRCA1* and *BRCA2* account for only a small percent of overall cases of breast cancer, but if you do happen to have one of these mutations you have a much higher risk of developing breast or ovarian cancer later in life. The final group of mutations are rare and only give a small risk of developing a disease (lower left). There are few examples of these types of mutations because they are hard to find.

Most of the common variants that greatly increase the chance of developing a disorder have already been found and as noted above, it is very difficult to find rare mutations that only slightly increase your risk of having a disease. Therefore, most research focuses on identifying either *common mutations of low risk (lower right) or rare mutations of high risk (upper left)*. An easy way to visualize the difference in these two categories is to think about getting cut by a pane of glass that suddenly falls to the ground and shatters. You would probably be fine with a few small cuts by slivers of flying glass, but if you had enough small cuts it might cause enough blood loss to put your life in danger. It all depends on the number of small injuries you sustain. On the other hand, if you are unlucky enough to be right next to the falling pane, you might be impaled by a single large shard of glass that would cause serious damage. In this case, the question is not how many cuts you receive, but whether you get the one large stab wound that is life threatening. This same logic can be used to determine your genetic risk of inheriting a disease. You can either look at how many common, low-risk mutations a person inherits (the slivers), or you can look to see if a patient inherits one or two rare, high-risk mutations (the shards).

The methods to find a genetic variant differ widely depending on if one is looking for slivers or shards. In order to find the slivers (common, low-risk mutations), researchers use a technique called genome-wide association studies. In a genome-wide association study, a researcher looks at the entire length of the DNA. Across all the DNA, some areas are almost identical in all people (these are called conserved regions), but other regions differ greatly between people (the variable regions). Say, for instance, there is one DNA nucleotide in the middle of chromosome 1 that is a 'G' in 90% of the population (this is called the major allele) and a 'T' in 10% of the population (this is called the minor allele). You can then ask the question of whether a person with the 'G' or a person with the 'T' is more likely to have a certain disease, such as attention deficit hyperactivity disorder (ADHD). In the early days of genetic research, this had to be done one at a time, but now with automation and more powerful computers, this process can be replicated millions of times across the entire genome in thousands of DNA samples, giving an unbiased look into which genetic variants increase the risk of a disease (the mutations) and which have no effect (normal variations).

The primary issue with genome-wide association studies is that each individual genetic mutation only gives a very small amount of risk. Because each individual effect is small, it takes thousands or tens of thousands of cases to find a difference. For example, a genome-wide association study might show that 14% of the general population has a 'T' nucleotide at a certain position, while 14.1% of patients with ADHD have a 'T' nucleotide at that position. So, while the T mutation may increase your risk of having ADHD, most people with the mutation will never have the illness.

Common, low risk variants also tend to be in the parts of the DNA far away from the protein-producing genes (only about 1% of your DNA is composed of the genes that encode proteins), so it can be difficult to tell how exactly the mutation increases risk of a disease because it is probably working on a gene far away from it (the regions of the DNA in between genes contain information on where, when, and how much of the protein that a gene encodes should be made, which is still poorly understood). A different set of methods are used to find the *shards* or the rare, high-risk mutations. I will go into detail on how to find these mutations in a later section.

<u>Original Sin</u>

The central problem of psychiatry research is that the Diagnostic and Statistical Manual lumped everyone with broadly similar features together even if they had different underlying causes of their symptoms.

Psychiatry researchers have continued down this path by using tools like functional MRI scanning and genome-wide association studies. Put another way, psychiatry continues to focus on *how groups of patients with a diagnosis are the same instead of how individual patients are unique.* Brain imaging studies scan groups of 20+ people to identify brain regions that are affected by an illness. Genetic studies lump thousands or tens of thousands of patients with the same diagnosis together. Medication trials still mainly focus on testing patients based upon Diagnostic and Statistical Manual criteria, because it is more profitable to do so, even though those criteria are not reliable. It should not be a surprise, then, that only small subsets of patients respond to our treatments (which were mostly discovered by serendipity).

Let's go back to our example from the first chapter. Imagine if we still lumped all patients with chest pain, shortness of breath, and fatigue into the diagnosis of chest pain syndrome. Now, imagine if you were trying to discover a new treatment for chest pain syndrome. If you gave everyone antibiotics, then the patients with bacterial pneumonia would get better, but it won't work for anyone else. If you tried using blood thinners, then patients with heart attacks and pulmonary embolisms would get better, patients with pneumonia would not get better, and patients with aortic dissection would probably die because it would increase bleeding. A tension pneumothorax requires a drainage tube to be placed, but this treatment would not help any of the other patients. In each case, arriving at a right diagnosis is the key to finding the right treatment. <u>*The key to improving treatments then is to identify factors that cause depression in individuals and design specific treatments for those patients.*</u>

Chapter 6: Precision Psychiatry

In the previous chapter, I discussed how psychiatry had erred in focusing too much on finding things in common between psychiatric diagnoses instead of identifying smaller groups of patients who share a common cause for their illness. But what does that look like in practice? How do you go about finding the root causes of a mental illness and then crafting individual treatments? In this chapter, I will present the concept of precision psychiatry and discuss how it is being used to answer questions like this.

Precision psychiatry is an off shoot of a larger movement called <u>precision medicine,</u> or sometimes personalized medicine. According to the Precision Medicine Initiative[42], the goal of precision medicine is to use "individual variability in genes, environment, and lifestyle[43]" to identify better ways to prevent and treat diseases. Concepts of precision medicine have circulated through the medical field for centuries, but really took off after the completion of the Human Genome Project in the early 2000s[44]. The goal of the Human Genome Project was to sequence all the DNA in the human chromosomes, and it provided a huge leap forward in the ability of researchers and clinicians to identify underlying genetic factors that cause diseases. Perhaps the best example of a precision medicine approach is in the field of <u>oncology.</u> Clinicians are now able to use genetic sequencing in certain types of cancer to identify mutated genes that affect specific pathways in cells that either cause the cell to grow uncontrollably or to not be able to be killed, and then develop specific treatments that target those pathways[45].

Precision medicine changed from being a movement in medicine to being more fully recognized as an individual field of study in 2015 when the Precision Medicine Initiative was announced by the National Institute of Health[46] and funded by Congress the following year. If, broadly speaking, the goal of evidenced-based practice is to find the best treatment *on average* for a group of people, then the goal of precision medicine is to find the best *specific* treatment for an individual person.

Precision psychiatry is far less developed as a field than precision medicine, although psychoanalytic psychotherapists would likely argue that they have been pursuing a form of highly individualized treatment since the work of Sigmund Freud. The term precision psychiatry first began being used in the mid-2010s[47], but has mostly remained isolated to academic settings where there are now several Departments of Psychiatry with precision psychiatry programs[48][49][50], an annual conference[51], and a textbook[52]. There are a few limited applications currently available for clinical practice, like the use of genetic testing to identify which psychiatric medications are more likely to work for a person with fewer side effects[53], but these tests still largely focus on the use of already known psychiatric medications instead of finding new treatments that may work better.

There will undoubtedly be many ways to accomplish this goal eventually. I have focused mostly on genetic approaches, but researchers now have ways of testing multiple different biological systems, including changes that affect the production of mRNA from genes (epigenomics), changes that affect the transcription of mRNA into proteins (transcriptomics), changes in the amounts of proteins in a cell (proteomics), changes in levels of small molecules in the cell (metabolomics), and changes in the level of lipids in the cell (lipidomics)[54]. For instance, we know that environmental factors like childhood trauma greatly increase the risk of later developing a mental illness[55]. But we also know that environmental factors do not increase the risk of mental illness by causing mutations in your DNA, so it is likely that environmental stressors work through one of these other pathways.

For the remainder of this book, though, I will focus on my approach, which has been to use genetics but with a slightly different focus than previous researchers and clinicians. As mentioned before, genetic mutations that cause diseases can be broadly thought of as either commonly found in the population but of low-risk (the slivers) or rarely found in the population but giving a high-risk (the shards). Most of the research has been done on these 'slivers' as I noted before, but how much of the risk of developing a psychiatric diagnosis is due to these common but low risk mutations? The answer to that question can be estimated from data in <u>genome-wide association studies</u>. The numbers range from a low of about 15% in autism to 43% in schizophrenia, while major depression, bipolar disorder, attention deficit hyperactivity disorder, and anorexia nervosa are all around 30%[56]. Put simply, most of the genetic risk for developing a psychiatric disorder does not come from common but low risk mutations (the 'slivers'). In order to fully understand how your genetics, affect your risk of developing a mental illness, we have to better understand the rare but high-risk mutations (the 'shards').

For a long time, it was very difficult to find the 'shards' because of the sheer amount of information held in your DNA— over 6 billion letters in total in each person. To put that in perspective, an average book page can hold around 1,500 letters on a single page. That means it would take a book more than 800 volumes with 500 pages each to hold all the information included in the DNA contained in each nucleus within every cell of your body. Because rare mutations are largely unknown, it means that you must analyze all the DNA in order to find them.

Initially, this cost was prohibitively expensive, but in recent years the price of sequencing DNA has dropped significantly, making it more widely accessible. The cost of sequencing an entire genome (all the DNA) is now less than $1,000 per person, and the cost of an exome (the 1% of your DNA covering just the protein-encoding genes) is less than $500.

Now that we can access all this information, the bigger problem has become how to understand all of it. I personally look at whole exome data because I am interested in mutations that change proteins, but even here the typical patient will have over 150,000 single nucleotide changes alone.

In the past, the most common way to find rare, high-risk mutations was to use a family study. In this kind of study, you must find a large family with multiple members affected by a rare or uncommon illness. Family studies have been done for disorders like breast cancer, Parkinson's disease, and amyotrophic lateral sclerosis (ALS, or Lou Gehrig's disease). In large families like this, there is usually around a 50/50 chance that each member of the family will develop one of these disorders, which is much higher than in the general population. Because the risk is around 50%, it suggests that there is a mutation in a single gene being passed along through the generations and you have a 50/50 chance of inheriting that gene from your mother or father. Once you find a family like this, you can sequence their DNA and find out which mutations are shared by the family members with the illness (and ideally not in the family members without the illness). This approach is a very powerful method to find rare, high-risk mutations, but with the major drawback that it requires a large family with multiple family members affected by an illness. Each person one generation apart (parent-child, sibling-sibling) shares about 50% of their DNA. So, a mother and daughter who have the same illness still share ½ their DNA. With 20,000+ genes total you may need as many as 15+ affected family members to be able to definitively identify a single gene mutation that runs in a family, and there are not very many families like this around.

Because it is unusual to find diseases that run in large families like this, we had to devise a new way to identify the rare, high-risk mutations that increase the risk of developing an illness. To accomplish this goal, I worked with a human geneticist, Jake Michaelson, to find an alternative strategy. Jake found a way to predict how likely a given gene is to have a highly damaging genetic mutation using publicly available DNA sequencing databases for tens of thousands of patients. He could then compare the frequency of highly damaging mutations in the public database to a set of patients with a specific disorder (in this case an eating disorder). This allowed us to identify genes that were likely involved in the development of eating disorders without needing to have large families with multiple family members with an illness.

In 2017, we published our results for 93 patients with eating disorders[57]. In that paper, we report 245 genes in patients with binge-eating behaviors that are more likely to have rare, highly damaging mutations and another 145 genes in patients with restrictive-eating behaviors. While each list represents only around 1% of the overall number of genes in the body, both lists had much higher rates of genes for peptide neurotransmitters (also called neuropeptides).

Neurotransmitters are molecules that help send information from neurons to another cell, like muscle, heart, or other nerve cells (see illustration on next page). Most people have heard of several well-known neurotransmitters like dopamine and serotonin, which are special molecules that are made from amino acids, but there is a wide range of neurotransmitters all with different properties. Peptide neurotransmitters are a unique type of neurotransmitter that are made from short pieces of proteins that are created using instructions from the DNA in your genes. So, while there is no gene for 'dopamine' or 'serotonin,' there are genes with instructions on how to make the peptide neurotransmitters and therefore there are also mutations in these genes that can change how they are made.

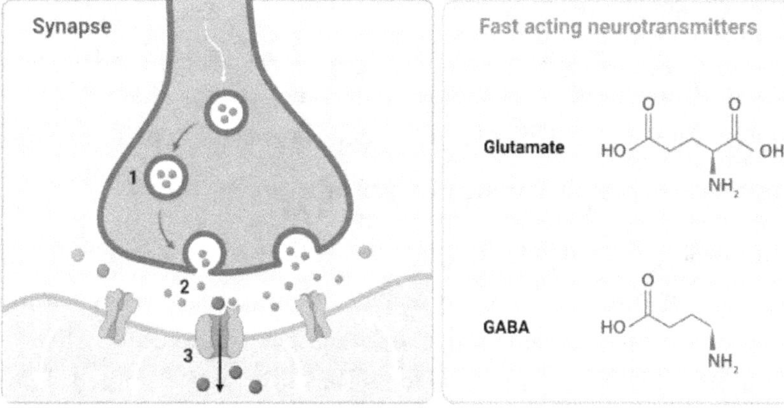

Neurotransmitters: neurons communicate by releasing chemical messengers called neurotransmitters. (1) When a neuron is activated, it releases small sacs filled with neurotransmitters called vesicles. (2) After being released from the neuron, the neurotransmitters float a short distance away to a neighboring cell where (3) it delivers its message by binding to a specific protein called a receptor.

Examples of different types of neurotransmitters: Fast acting neurotransmitters can activate neurons (glutamate) or inhibit neurons (GABA) (upper right). Monoamine neurotransmitters like dopamine, serotonin, and norepinephrine are common targets of psychiatric medications (middle). Peptide neurotransmitters like endorphins are made from amino acids using instruction from genes in the DNA (lower).

There are over 100 known neuropeptides in the body that affect a wide variety of processes, including sleep, pain tolerance, digestion, thirst, appetite, and body weight[58]. Probably the most famous neuropeptide is beta-endorphin, also commonly referred to as endorphins. Beta-endorphin is released during vigorous activity and is associated with the 'runner's high' that some individuals get after exercise, but it is also involved in regulating several functions including pain tolerance, sensitivity to rewarding things, and appetite, among others[59].

In retrospect, it is probably not that surprising that patients with eating disorders are more likely to have damaging mutations in genes involved in appetite, gut function, and body weight regulation, but when we discovered this, it was a very new idea. The initial study required almost 100 people in order to find genes with 'clusters' of mutations, so it was not very helpful for single individuals. However, it did provide insight into better understanding the factors that increase your risk of developing an eating disorder. It also gave a framework for helping to predict which genes were more likely to be mutated in patients with a certain disease.

A good example of this are the mutations we reported for a neuropeptide called glucagon-like peptide 1 or GLP-1. Glucagon-like peptide 1 is a peptide hormone/neurotransmitter that is made from the glucagon gene. The glucagon gene encodes a long peptide chain that is then further broken down into several smaller peptides including glucagon and glucagon-like peptide 1. Glucagon is expressed in the pancreas next to the cells that make insulin and mainly acts to counter the effects of insulin by increasing glucose levels when your blood sugar is low. Unlike glucagon, glucagon-like peptide 1 is made primarily in the small intestine and in the brain, where it is released after eating. Glucagon-like peptide 1 released from the intestines has several actions to help with the digestion of food, including slowing the release of food from the stomach, stimulating the release of insulin from the pancreas, and helping insulin work better. In the brain, glucagon-like peptide 1 affects regions involved in satiety and reward to help a person feel satisfied and stop eating during a meal.

Of the 55 people in the study who struggled with binge eating, four of them had mutations in the glucagon-like peptide 1 system. All four of these individuals also struggled with self-induced vomiting as well. The fact that glucagon-like peptide 1 is expressed in both the gut and the brain may help explain this observation. In the brain, glucagon-like peptide 1 makes you feel full and satisfied and in the gut, it helps with digestion and the storage of nutrients. Patients who lack glucagon-like peptide 1 describe eating to the point of being physically uncomfortable, but still feeling hungry, possibly because the brain does not get a signal that food is present, and the gut has a hard time digesting the food. Many patients report the unpleasant experience of feeling physically distended but still being hungry and feeling like they should continue to eat. The only way to relieve this disconnect between the mind and the body is through self-induced vomiting.

Private Mutations

A private mutation refers to a change in the DNA that occurs in only a single individual or a small family. In addition to my own work, an increasing number of research studies are finding that private mutations contribute to the risk of developing psychiatric disorders including bipolar disorder[60], schizophrenia[61], autism[62], and obsessive-compulsive disorder[63]. As mentioned above, if you look at all the mutations in a large group of patients with a certain illness, patterns begin to emerge. Certain genes are much more likely to be mutated in specific diseases. For instance, people with schizophrenia frequently have a mutation in a group of ten genes that are related to connections between neurons called synapses[64], but there is a catch. Just because we know that *some* mutations in a certain gene can increase your risk of developing an illness, that does not mean that *all* mutations in a gene increase your risk. Genes are thousands of letters long, and mutations can occur at any of those thousands of positions. Critically, the effects of a change in one of these letters can be very dependent on where it occurs within the gene. Take the *BRCA1* and *BRCA2* genes, for example. These genes are sometimes called the "breast cancer genes" because many mutations in them have been associated with an increased risk of certain cancers, including breast and ovarian cancers[65]. However, if you look at all the mutations that have been found in the BRCA1 gene[66], you find that some clearly increase your risk of cancer, some clearly don't increase your risk, and in many cases, it is unclear if the mutations increase your risk or not.

Many of these uncertain mutations are rare or private mutations and therefore present their own set of challenges. As discussed earlier, most genetic studies look at how common a mutation is in a group of patients with a disease versus how common they are in a control group of individuals without the disease. This approach is impossible to do with a private mutation because there are not enough people with the mutation to make a comparison (unless you have a large family, which is a rare occurrence). For example, a patient may have a private mutation in *BRCA1* and develop breast cancer. Around 70% of patients with disease-causing mutations in *BRCA1* will develop cancer in their lifetime, but about 13% of *all* women in the United States will develop breast cancer in their lifetime[67], so it is impossible to tell *in a single case* if the mutation caused the cancer or if it was just a coincidence.

This problem of private mutations will be a central focus in modern psychiatry. We know that rare or private mutations in certain genes are important in causing psychiatric illness, but we don't yet have the tools to determine which mutations increase the risk of a disease and which have little or no effect. Moreover, in the case of psychiatric disorders, some mutations may cause or exacerbate some symptoms of a disease but have little or no effect on other symptoms. The entire biomedical system and the idea of evidence-based practice is designed around clustering people into large groups that can be carefully tested. Many common research methods can't even be conducted on a single individual, including functional brain scans and randomized controlled clinical trials. While certain diseases may share some symptoms in common (like suicidal thoughts, hallucinations, or compulsive behaviors), there is not a system in place to study a disease process that occurs in a single person or family. In the next few chapters, we will examine what it looks like to treat a person with a private mutation by focusing on patients with eating disorders, which is one of the fields that I specialize in. What are the challenges that must be overcome to truly personalize medicine? What new methods for research and treatment will have to be developed? What can be done now to provide better treatments?

Chapter 7: Anorexia Nervosa

Anorexia nervosa remains one of the most poorly understood illnesses in medicine. The two major symptoms of anorexia, distortion of body image and fear of eating, seem to be completely opposed to our normal survival instincts. In this chapter, I will present the use of precision psychiatry approaches to understand an enigmatic illness.

Anorexia nervosa has one of the most straightforward diagnostic criteria of all the mental illnesses in the Diagnostic and Statistical Manual of Mental Disorders, and yet it also remains one of the most poorly understood. In the fifth edition of the manual there are only three criteria[68]:

1. Restriction of energy intake relative to requirements, leading to a significant low body weight in the context of the age, sex, developmental trajectory, and physical health (less than minimally normal/expected).
2. Intense fear of gaining weight or becoming fat or persistent behavior that interferes with weight gain.
3. Disturbed by one's body weight or shape, self-worth influenced by body weight or shape, or persistent lack of recognition of seriousness of low bodyweight.

Anorexia can be further categorized into two subtypes. 'Binge-eating/purging type' occurs when a patient also engages in episodes of binge eating and/or purging behaviors. Binging is characterized by recurrent episodes of uncontrollably eating large amounts of food, while purging refers to any efforts to eliminate food from your system before it can be absorbed[69]. 'Restricting type' occurs when there is only restriction and no repeated episodes of binging or purging[70].

While the diagnostic criteria of anorexia nervosa are relatively straightforward, the underlying causes of the disorder have remained elusive. We do know for certain that the risk of developing anorexia is a combination of genetic risk factors and environmental stressors. Eating disorders are much more likely to run in families (a person with anorexia is five times more likely to have a close family member with anorexia than you would expect by chance). Environmental stressors can then trigger eating disorder behaviors in people who have this underlying genetic vulnerability. While the genetic mutations that increase the risk of developing anorexia are largely unknown, the environmental triggers are much better understood, including things like trauma, pressures to be thin/lose weight, and medical illnesses that cause malnourishment.

I won't go into detail on the environmental triggers for anorexia here (there are much better books for that). Instead, I will focus on biological factors that increase the risk of developing an eating disorder. Specifically, I will present the use of whole exome sequencing to identify the genetic mutations that increase the risk of anorexia and how we can use that information to improve treatments. Whole exome sequencing gives us a picture of all the protein-encoding regions of all the genes in the genome. The primary benefit of whole exome sequencing is that it is what we call an unbiased approach because it looks at all 20,000+ genes instead of narrowing in on a few that we think are most likely to be important. Put another way, this technique removes the bias of looking at specific genes, which is critical when we have no preconceived idea of which gene mutations might be causing the risk.

A good analogy for an unbiased approach would be a murder investigation. In this example, a person is found to have been murdered and the investigators must figure out who committed the crime. A traditional investigation might focus on a few people close to the victim and try to rule them in or out as the murderer. An alternative approach would be to take a piece of evidence like a fingerprint on the crime scene and then try to find a match for it. The traditional approach is considered 'biased' because the investigators have focused on a small group of suspects and have a strong incentive to find the murderer among the people that they investigate, even if the evidence is inconclusive. The second approach is considered 'unbiased' because it looks at every individual capable of being the murderer without excluding any potential suspects.

Science experiments are similar to murder investigations. Narrowing in on a few likely suspects may be easier and less expensive, but it can often decrease the objectivity of the research. A good example of this comes from the field of major depression research. For years it was too expensive to sequence all the genes in a patient's DNA, so researchers had to use what was called the candidate gene approach. In the candidate gene approach, researchers would make educated guesses on which genes were most likely to cause a disease and then look for mutations only in those genes (i.e., the likely suspects). Many depression researchers initially focused on genes involving serotonin because most antidepressant medications work by increasing serotonin levels. These experiments did lead to some interesting findings on how people with depression respond to antidepressant medications, but they did not find out much about the actual causes of depression, because it turns out that lack of serotonin does not cause most cases of depression. Going back to our analogy of a murder investigation, scientists spent years trying to prove that low serotonin levels cause major depression in much the same way that an investigator might focus for too long on trying to prove the lover of the murder victim is the killer.

In contrast, unbiased scientific experiments (like whole exome sequencing) tend to be more difficult and more expensive to do, but they give better results because any findings that are made could be important no matter what is discovered. Unbiased experiments also tend to be more objective, because there is no incentive to fit data to the initial hypothesis. In the analogy of a murder investigation, this would be the equivalent of finding a match for the fingerprint found at the crime scene in the database. No matter who the person is, if you find their fingerprint on a murder victim then the result is important to the investigation.

One of the most striking things about unbiased approaches is that the results are often completely unexpected, so you would never find them only by taking an educated guess. Anorexia is a good example of a completely unexpected result. I have now sequenced the genes of hundreds of patients with eating disorders, and the results for anorexia are as clear to me as they are striking. While I have found several different subtypes of anorexia, *the most common issue I have found is that patients with anorexia are much more likely to have damaging mutations in genes involved in storing body fat and burning it for energy.* At first, this idea seems ridiculous. One popular idea is that obesity is caused by the inability to burn fat, with many 'miracle fat burning cures' marketed for weight loss. Patients with anorexia have very low body fat, so if anything, the prevailing wisdom would predict that they burn fat too well. To better appreciate what goes wrong in anorexia, it is first helpful to understand how the body responds to fasting.

In order to demonstrate how the body adapts to periods of fasting, let's use the analogy of a factory with a large wood-burning furnace. A full animated version of the video is available at:

www.Precision-Psychiatry.com/video[1]

If you are not able to watch the video currently, a series of images from the video are shown on the following pages with descriptions.

---

1. http://www.Precision-Psychiatry.com/video

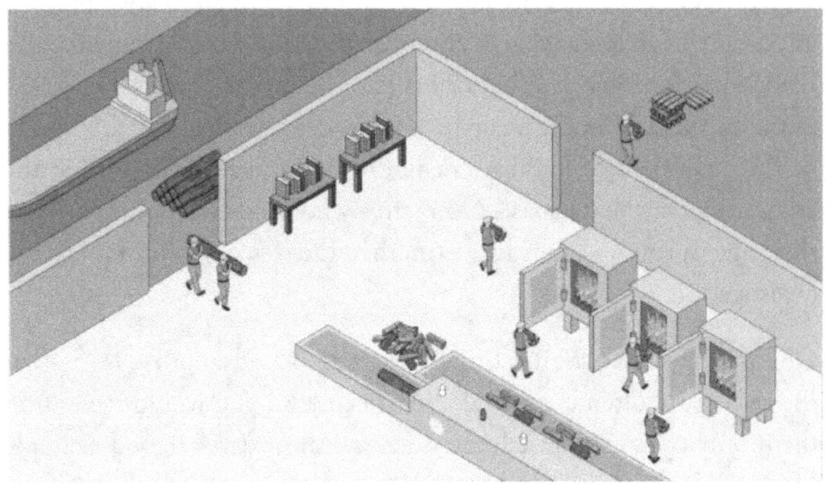

Imagine that this factory sits on the edge of a river. Throughout the factory there are several large furnaces that burn wood to produce energy to run the factory (lower right corner of the illustration). Each day three large boats bring in shipments of trees (upper left corner). The workers unload these different types of wood and cut them into logs small enough to put into the furnace to burn for energy. Sometimes when the shipments of wood are really large, there are extra logs which can be taken outside, wrapped up into big bundles, and stored in a large pile behind the factory to use later (upper right corner).

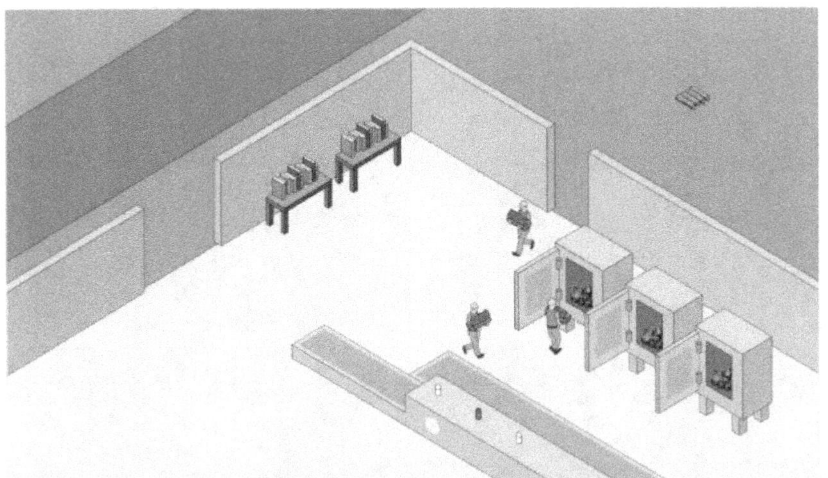

Now let's imagine what happens when all of a sudden, the boats stop coming in to deliver shipments of trees? The factory workers will quickly run out of logs and the fire will start to cool down (lower right corner). The first thing that the workers can do is bring in the extra logs that were stored outside the factory (upper right corner).

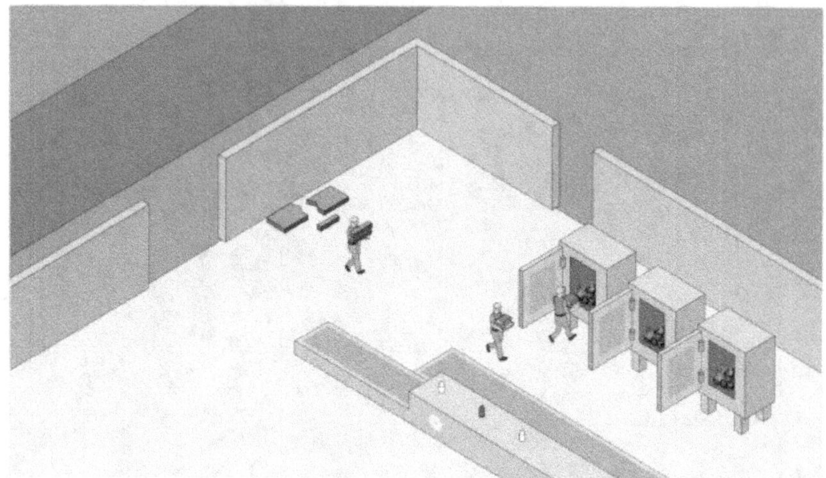

Let's take things one step further and imagine that the supply of stored logs starts to run out. As the furnace starts to cool and energy starts to run low again, there is one more option to keep the fire burning. The workers can take pieces of wood that are laying around the factory like books and furniture (center of illustration) and burn that for energy until, eventually, everything they can possibly burn is used up.

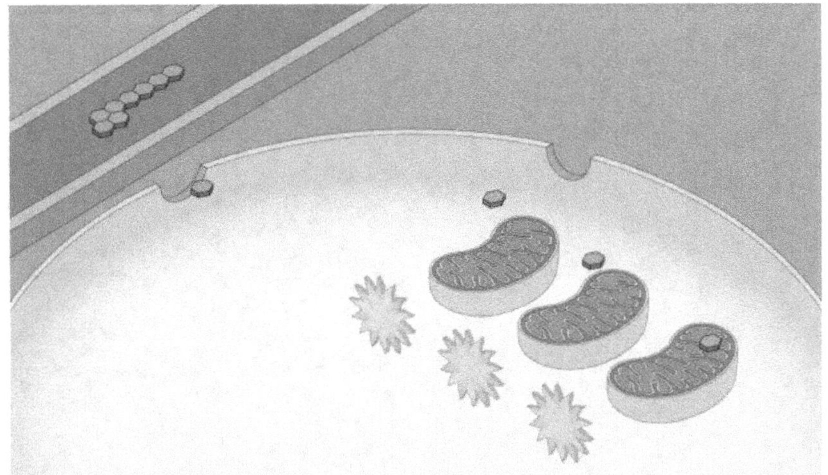

The analogy of the factory is similar to how the cells in your body function. The factory represents a cell in the body and the furnaces represent a part of the cell called the <u>mitochondria</u> (the kidney bean-shaped images in the lower right corner). Mitochondria take nutrients from the food that is eaten and turn it into energy that the cells can use to function in the same way that a furnace burns wood to create energy to run the factory (energy is shown as yellow sun-shaped bursts next to the mitochondria). The shipments of trees represent different carbohydrates that come from the food that you eat (brown hexagons in the upper left corner). Carbohydrates are nutrients that can be broken down into glucose, a type of fuel that the mitochondria can easily use to produce energy.

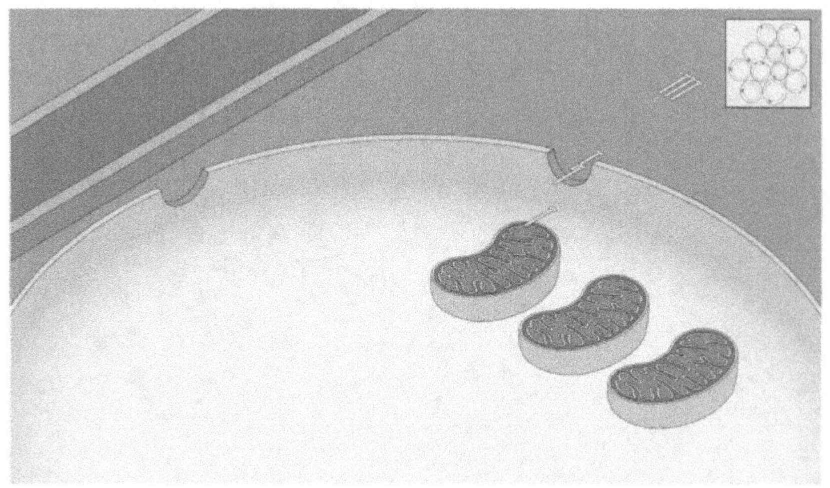

The extra logs that are bundled up for later use represent <u>fatty acids</u> that the body stores in fat cells (yellow T-shapes coming from the fat cells in the upper right corner). During a prolonged fast, the body does not have enough glucose and has to switch to stored nutrients like fat for energy.

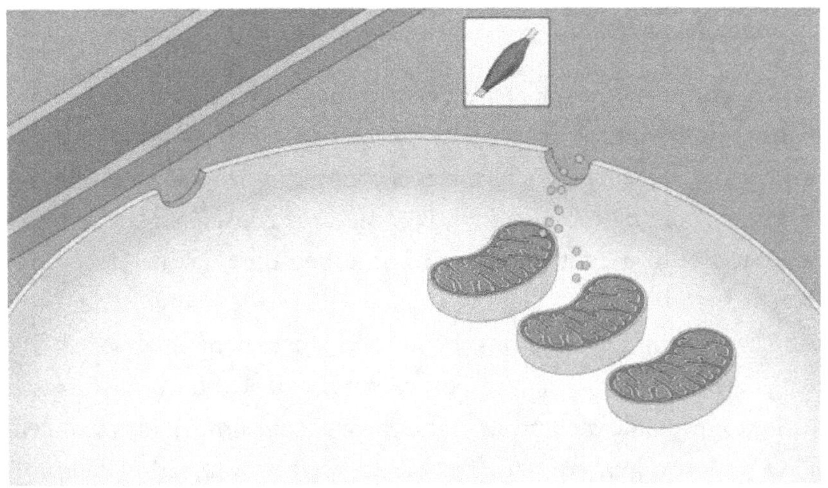

In extreme cases, the body can start breaking down proteins like muscle and connective tissue in order to get amino acids to use as energy (muscle is the upper center of the illustration and amino acids are shown as purple spheres moving into the mitochondria).

<u>Errors in metabolism</u>

As I mentioned above, I have come to believe that anorexia nervosa is the result of not being able to burn fatty acids and certain amino acids from proteins. This idea seems counterintuitive at first. Obesity, a state of holding too much fat, is commonly considered the result of an inability to use fat for energy. For a long time, I was reluctant to accept the idea as well, but eventually, when patient after patient had similar patterns of mutations, I could no longer deny the science. The data have forced me to accept a different view of how the body works in order to reconcile the findings. The theory that I now hold is that cells have ways to signal back to the brain to change your eating behaviors and your metabolism depending on which nutrients your body can use as fuel for energy production. We currently view all nutrients as the same: carbohydrates, proteins, and fats can all be broken down equally by the cell for energy. But what if, in the process of breaking down those nutrients, the cell signals back to the brain to change what type of foods to eat or avoid? In order to better understand this, it might be helpful to understand in more detail how fat and protein (the body reserves for energy) are broken down and turned into energy.

Fat is stored in adipose cells as a triglyceride, which is composed of 3 separate fatty acids linked together. <u>Fatty acids</u> themselves are large chains of carbons usually in an even number. Short chain fatty acids contain between 2 to 6 carbons, medium chain fatty acids contain 6 to 12 carbons, long chain fatty acids contain 13 to 21 carbons, and very long chain fatty acids contain 22 or more carbons. Fatty acids link together to form <u>triglycerides</u>, which can be a very effective way to store energy, but it does take some effort in order to pull the fatty acids out of storage and be converted into energy. The triglycerides must be broken down into individual fatty acids, then transported in the blood throughout the body where they are taken up by cells. Fatty acids that are less than 13 carbons long can just move into the <u>mitochondria</u> on their own to be turned into energy, but long chain fatty acids are too big to just move into the mitochondria on their own, so there is an entire process that has evolved to shuttle long chain fatty acids into the mitochondria. It starts by linking the long chain fatty acid to a molecule called <u>carnitine</u>. This combined carnitine-long chain fatty acid molecule can now be moved into the center of the mitochondria using a special transport system[71]. Once inside the mitochondria, the long chain fatty acids are broken down two carbons at a time and used to make more energy for the cell. Patients with anorexia are more likely to mutations in genes related to making carnitine like *BBOX* and transporting carnitine-long chain fatty acid molecules into the mitochondria like *CPT1* and *CPT2*.

The second reserve source of fuel that your cells can use for energy is to break down proteins into amino acids. As mentioned before, there are 20 different amino acids that your body uses to make proteins and each one of them can also be broken down and used as fuel by the mitochondria to turn into energy. I won't detail the step-by-step process of each one, but as a representative example, I will go through the process of breaking down three amino acids called valine, leucine, and isoleucine, which are also known as the branched chain amino acids (BCAAs). The first step in the process involves a protein called the Branched Chain Aminotransferase, which removes the 'amine' part of the amino acid, leaving it as something called a ketoacid. The second step in the process involves a group of proteins called the Branched Chain Keto Acid Dehydrogenase, which basically removes the 'acid' part of the original amino acid and releases it as carbon dioxide. From here, additional steps can be taken to complete the process of turning all three of the branched chain amino acids into molecules that the mitochondria can turn into energy.

People with anorexia are more likely to have damaging mutations in genes that make the proteins involved in breaking down <u>long chain fatty acids</u> and <u>essential amino acids</u> into energy than people who do not have anorexia, especially this subset of amino acids called branched-chain amino acids. From this observation, I developed a theory that patients with anorexia are more likely to have difficulty breaking down certain fats and proteins for energy when they are fasting, which leads to a build-up of these molecules. *This accumulation of fatty acids and branched chain amino acids act as a signal back to the brain to change your appetite and this is ultimately what triggers the strong aversion to eating, especially to calorically dense foods like fat and meat.*

<u>Nutrient Sensing Pathways</u>

For this theory to be correct, there must be a pathway within the cell that senses the presence of available nutrients. This same pathway would also have to be able to send a signal to the brain to control your appetite, specifically telling the brain not to eat certain foods that your cells can not break down and use as fuel.

For a long time, I struggled with identifying what this pathway could be. There are several known energy sensors for things like glucose, amino acids, and fatty acids throughout the body, but it was not clear to me which specific pathway(s) could be responsible for sensing the build-up of nutrients and telling the brain to change eating behaviors. The key piece to the puzzle came one day when I was doing an analysis of patients with both seizures and anorexia. This specific group of patients was more likely to have damaging mutations in two genes called *DEPDC5* and *TSC2*. These two genes are part of a pathway known as <u>mTOR</u>[72]. The mTOR pathway is a well-known regulator of cell growth and survival. One of the ways that it determines whether a cell should grow is by sensing the presence of nutrients like fatty acids[73] and essential amino acids, including arginine and branched-chain amino acids like leucine[74]. In this way, mTOR makes sure the body has enough energy and nutrients available for cells to grow and divide. If mTOR senses that there are not enough nutrients available, it tells the cells to stop growing and conserve energy.

Even more importantly, though, is the fact that there is some evidence that mTOR regulates food intake, at least in mice anyway. When you turn on mTOR in mice in a part of the brain known to regulate food intake (the mediobasal hypothalamus), it suppresses food intake and body weight[17]. When you combine the fact that mTOR is activated by excess fatty acids and amino acids, and that activated mTOR suppresses food intake and lowers body weight, it suggests that mTOR might be the critical link between impaired metabolism of fat and proteins and the behavior changes seen in anorexia.

Let's return to the images from the animation to illustration these points.

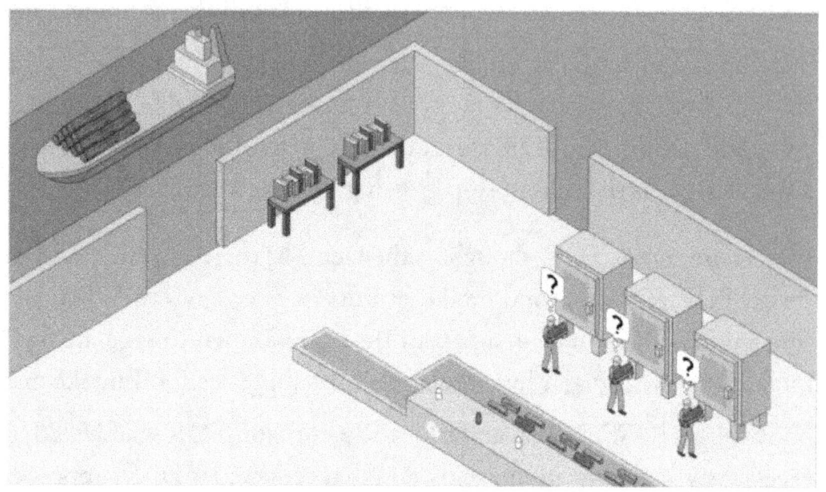

People with anorexia respond differently to periods of fasting though. Let's go back to the analogy of the factory. Imagine that there is something wrong with the door to the furnace and the workers are not able to open it to put the wood on the fire to burn (lower right corner). The logs are still brought to the furnace, but now they start to pile up on the factory floor instead of being used to fuel the furnace.

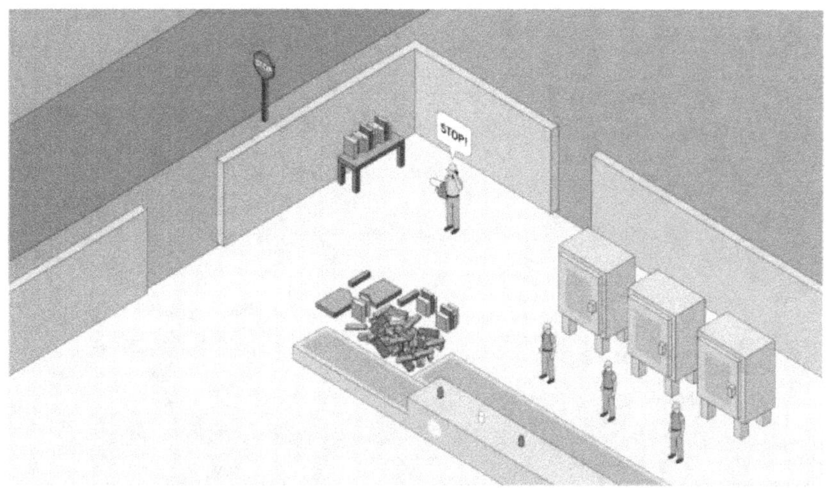

A supervisor comes in and sees the logs and pieces of broken furniture piling up on the floor (center). The supervisor mistakenly believes that there is plenty of fuel available and cancels any further shipments of wood.

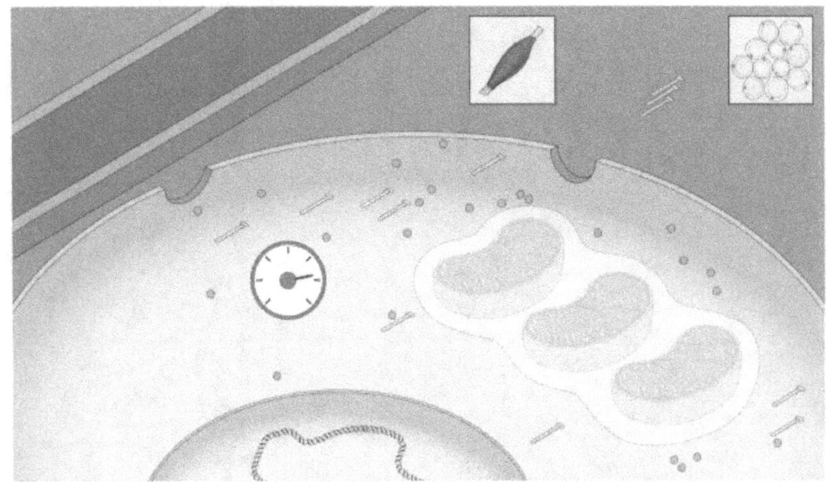

Something like this is what I think happens in anorexia. Certain individuals inherit rare, highly damaging mutations in genes related to using fat and protein for energy (represented by the gray covering or the mitochondria in the lower right corner). A person can do fine as long as they are eating regularly and there is not a huge increase in the demand for energy. However, the system cannot keep up whenever food intake decreases, or the body suddenly needs more energy. As a result, amino acids (purple spheres) and fatty acids (yellow T-shapes) start to build up within the cell.

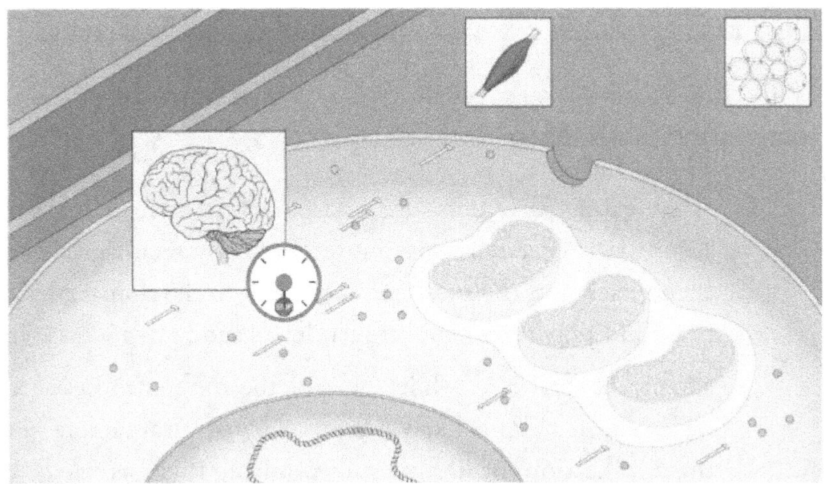

In this example, the supervisor acts like mTOR, and like the supervisor, mTOR senses the presence of long-chain fatty acids (yellow T-shapes) and essential amino acids (purple spheres) and incorrectly concludes that there is an abundance of nutrients. As a result of this incorrect conclusion, mTOR then sends out a message that there are too many nutrients leading to a strong aversion to eating (the full gas gauge with the red stop sign).

While this theory is unexpected, if true, it does potentially answer some lingering questions in the field:

1. Why eating disorders are more common in females— Anorexia is over ten times more frequently seen in females than males, and the most common time to develop anorexia is around puberty when estrogen levels suddenly increase in adolescent girls[75]. While some of the difference between males and females is likely explained by cultural factors like the idealization of thinness in women, there is likely a biological component as well. Estrogen suppresses appetite and estrogen receptors are expressed in the same region of the brain that regulates appetite (the <u>mediobasal hypothalamus</u>) that we have already discussed[76]. Furthermore, the nutrient sensor mTOR is required for estrogen to suppress appetite (at least in mice)[77]. One possible explanation is that the rapid increase in estrogen levels at puberty causes the appetite suppressing region of the brain to be much more sensitive by increasing mTOR activity.

2. Fear of fat— The diagnostic criteria for anorexia merely require that an individual restricts their food intake, but we have long known that patients with anorexia have a specific aversion to fat[78] [79]. If my theory is true that many patients with anorexia have difficulty with breaking down fat for energy, then the build-up of long chain fatty acids in certain part of the brain that control appetite and body image may explain why individuals with anorexia have a specific aversion to dietary fat and a fear of becoming fat. It's the brains intuitive way of telling you not to depend on a source of

energy that it has a hard time using.

3. How negative energy states can trigger anorexia— We have long known that being in a negative energy state (taking in fewer calories than you consume) can trigger symptoms of anorexia, but we did not know how that process occurred. The most famous example of a negative energy state triggering anorexia is dieting to lose weight, but we know that several other situations can also trigger restriction urges, including participating in endurance sports and certain medical conditions that make it difficult to digest and absorb foods, especially gastrointestinal disorders. This theory suggests that patients with anorexia fail to respond appropriately to negative energy states, because fasting releases stored nutrients like fatty acids from triglycerides and amino acids from proteins that the <u>mitochondria</u> in the cells cannot efficiently use for energy. *The brain inappropriately sees the build-up of these fatty acids or amino acids as a sign of nutritional excess and turns off the appetite.* Patients then enter a spiral where they eat less and less food which causes the release of more fatty acids and more amino acids, which causes further weight loss.

4. The link between anxiety, seizures, and anorexia— Researchers and clinicians have long appreciated that patients with anorexia often (but not always) have similar personality features. They tend to be very anxious, perfectionistic, low risk taking, and struggle with adapting to change. Up to two-thirds of patients with anorexia meet the criteria for diagnosis of an anxiety disorder[80]. Patients with anorexia also tend to have an increased risk of having a seizure[81]. Both anxiety disorders and seizures have been linked to disruptions in the neurotransmitter GABA in the brain[82] [83]. GABA is the primary inhibitory neurotransmitter in the brain, which

means that GABA stops other neurons from firing. Medications that increase GABA signaling in the brain are used in a wide variety of conditions in which you need to slow down the activity of neurons, including anxiety, seizures, and insomnia. Could mTOR explain the link between all three? Epilepsy researchers have already shown that mTOR increases the risk of having a seizure by affecting GABA signaling in the brain[84], so it is possible that increased mTOR activity could explain both the eating disorder symptoms and the anxiety symptoms we see in patients with anorexia as well.

5. How trauma triggers anorexia— In addition to regulating food intake, the mediobasal hypothalamus is also an important site in how the body responds to stress. Two smaller areas of the mediobasal hypothalamus, the dorsomedial nucleus of the hypothalamus and the ventromedial nucleus of the hypothalamus, are involved in physical responses to psychological stress including changes in heart rate, blood pressure, and body temperature[85]. Therefore, two well-known risk factors for anorexia, stress and estrogen, both affect the same region of the brain (see illustration on next page).

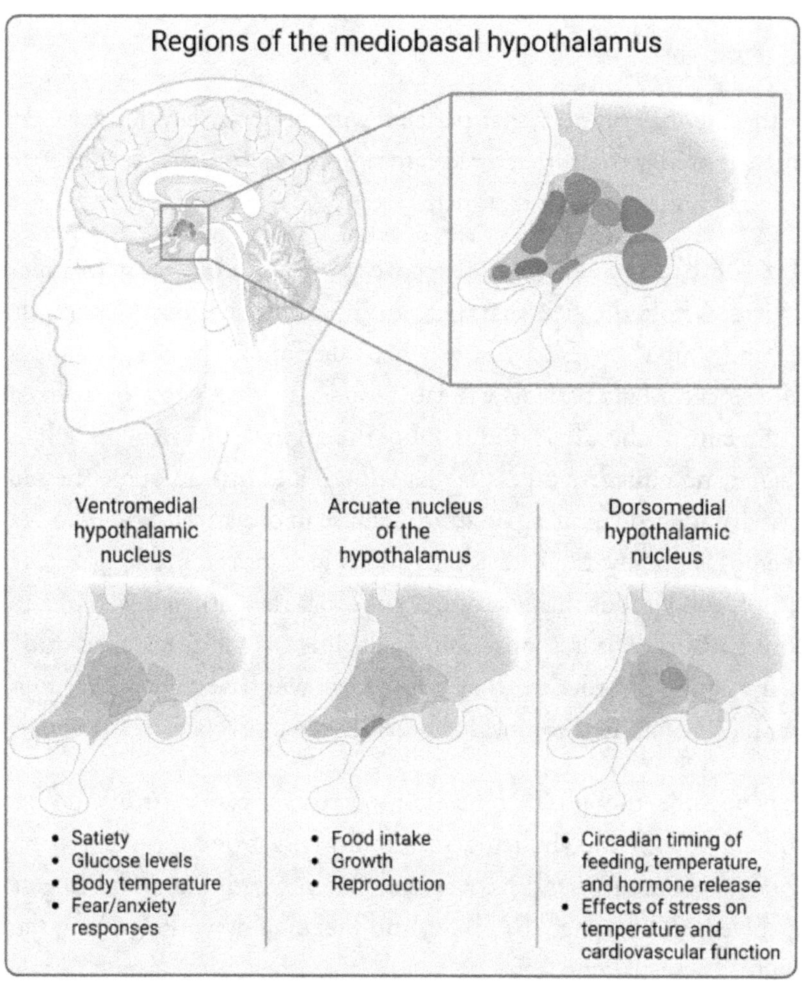

Regions of the mediobasal hypothalamus
Ventromedial hypothalamic nucleus
Arcuate nucleus of the hypothalamus
Dorsomedial hypothalamic nucleus
• Satiety
• Glucose levels
• Body temperature
• Fear/anxiety responses
• Food intake
• Growth
• Reproduction
• Circadian timing of feeding, temperature, and hormone release
• Effects of stress on temperature and cardiovascular function

<u>Implications</u>

If the theory is correct that patients with anorexia have impairments in their ability to utilize stored fat and protein for energy, then it has several implications for treatment:

The "no bad foods" model of recovery— Right now, most treatment providers hold the view that there are 'no bad foods.' Foods containing fat and simple sugars have largely been demonized by the anti-obesity movement. Many patients will label foods as either 'good' or 'bad' and begin cutting these 'bad' foods out of their diet. Other patients will feel shame and guilt around eating 'bad' foods and instead purge the food by self-induced vomiting or laxative abuse in order to rid their body of them. Eventually, the list of 'bad' foods gets longer and longer as the list of 'good' foods shrinks to the point that the patient develops a full eating disorder. In response to this labeling of 'good' and 'bad' foods, many eating disorder treatment providers will have patients eat foods containing fat, sugar, or meat as a standard part of their treatment.

It is possible, though, that a certain percent of patients really do have difficulty with metabolizing macronutrients from specific types of food. As noted earlier, I have several patients with mutations in genes involved in digesting, absorbing, and breaking down long-chain fatty acids. These patients tend to report that they need a much higher number of calories in order to gain weight compared to other similar patients at treatment centers, sometimes needing 4000-5000 calories per day to restore weight[86].

If it is true that some patients just don't break down certain nutrients very well, then it opens the possibility of creating meal plans tailored to specific individuals. For instance, certain meal plans may limit excess amounts of protein or foods high in long-chain fatty acids if a patient has a mutation that affects their ability to break that type of food down into energy. I find that many patients with mutations in genes related to breaking down essential amino acids report being vegetarian or vegan even before the onset of their eating disorder (plant proteins tend to have lower amounts of essential amino acids[87]). Individual meal plans are commonly designed for certain medical conditions like inborn errors of metabolism, but it is not common in the eating disorder field outside of eliminating gluten for patients with celiac disease. It would represent a significant departure from the current standard of treatment.

Setting treatment goals for patients— The standard goal of treatment centers has long been to achieve "ideal" body weight. I use the term "ideal" in quotation marks because the methods for determining a patient's ideal body weight have always been very controversial. In children and adolescents, dietitians at most eating disorder treatment centers use the patient's growth chart, if available, to set a target weight that basically puts them back on their original growth curve[88]. Once patients get to adulthood, the most common method is to use a simple equation called the <u>Hamwi formula</u> to calculate the "ideal" body weight. For women, that formula is 100 pounds + 5 pounds for every 1 inch above five feet in height. Most dietitians will then add a few pounds on either side of this number to create a weight range to account for normal fluctuations in weight. So, for a woman who is 5'4" the "ideal" body weight is 100 lb. + (4 inches X 5 pounds/inch above five feet) = 120 lb. The weight range might then be something like 115-125 lbs. or 118-122 lbs. depending on the preference of the dietitian. For a man, the formula is 106 lb. + 6 pounds for every inch of height above five feet tall. An alternative approach is to use the method of body mass index (<u>BMI</u>) with the goal of trying to stay in the 20-25 range for BMI.

These calculations are fraught with controversy though. The biggest challenge to this method is that the formulas were created with data collected mostly from the Metropolitan Life Insurance company in the 1940s and 1950s, which are not accurate reflections of the ethnic diversity in the United States or around the world[89]. The second concern is that the formulas predict that all people of the same height should be within a few pounds of weight to each other (the BMI method provides a slightly larger range of acceptable weights). This prediction clearly flies in the face of any observation of human diversity.

It's not clear to me that body weight goals set by eating disorder treatment programs benefit patients. From working with people over the years, I have gotten the clear message that weight based goals are not their preference. Most patients, unless they are severely underweight, report that what bothers them the most is the intense levels of shame and guilt they feel around what they eat and how they experience their body weight and shape. Treatment programs knowingly dismiss the wishes of their patients (to reduce eating disorder thoughts and body image distress) in order to meet the goals of insurance companies (to achieve 1-3 pounds of weight gain per week).

The current thinking is that patients with anorexia have become *afraid of the act of eating* and they must be exposed to this fear through aggressive re-feeding and learn to tolerate the distress. The genetic findings suggest quite a different possibility that refeeding makes eating disorder thoughts worse because patients with anorexia have difficulty with breaking down certain nutrients, which triggers anxiety responses through mTOR. Genetically informed approaches may someday allow us to recenter the focus of treatment on symptoms important to the patient, with body weight as a secondary goal of treatment.

Chapter 8: Other Pathways That Affect Eating Disorders

In the previous chapter, I went into detail on one specific pathway that appears to be related to the risk of developing anorexia, but this is just one pathway among several that seem to increase the risk of developing an eating disorder. This makes a lot of sense if you consider the broad range of symptoms that people with eating disorders exhibit. We have covered restriction of food intake and over-exercising, but there are many others including binging on large amounts of food, purging (by self-induced vomiting or laxative use), orthorexia (avoiding foods that one thinks are harmful), rumination (regurgitating food that has been swallowed and chewing on it again), night eating, fluid restriction, fear of choking/ gagging, and eating non-food items. In the next chapter, I will review some of the other pathways that I have found to be affected in patients with a variety of eating behaviors.

<u>Peptide neurotransmitters</u>

Earlier in this book, I presented the example of glucagon-like peptide 1. Glucagon-like peptide 1 is a hormone that is released by your intestines after you eat and has several functions, including stimulating insulin release (to help store glucose from your meal for later use as energy), and making you feel more satisfied after eating. Glucagon-like peptide 1 is one of many peptide neurotransmitters or <u>neuropeptides</u>, which means that it is a neurotransmitter that is made from a protein that is encoded by a gene. While mutations in glucagon-like peptide 1 mostly result in bulimia nervosa and binge eating disorder, there are several other peptide neurotransmitters that appear to be involved in the risk of developing eating disorders as well.

Beta-endorphin— Beta-endorphin, or just 'endorphins[90]' as it is more popularly called, is part of a subset of peptide neurotransmitters called the opioid peptides. Most people are more familiar with opioids that are used either as drugs of abuse (like heroin) or as medications (like morphine, oxycodone, and fentanyl, which can also be misused as drugs of abuse). These are sometimes referred to as exogenous (which means coming from the outside or external) opioids because they are made outside the body and consumed to produce their effect. There is also an endogenous (meaning inside or internal) opioid system that is produced by the body. The <u>endogenous opioid system</u> consists of several members, including beta-endorphin, as well as enkephalin and dynorphin[91]. The endogenous opioid system functions mainly to help the body counteract the effects of chronic stress by increasing pain tolerance, slowing breathing, improving mood, slowing the gastrointestinal tract, and increasing appetite.

Of the three endogenous opioid peptide neurotransmitters, endorphin, dynorphin, and enkephalin, the one that I see mutated most frequently in eating disorder patients is beta-endorphin. Beta-endorphin is made from a gene called *Proopiomelanocortin*. Like many other peptide neurotransmitters, the *Proopiomelanocortin* gene encodes information for a much longer protein that is then cut up into smaller peptide neurotransmitters. Depending on the body tissue in which pre-opiomelanocortin is expressed, it can be turned into adrenocorticotrophic hormone (which increases cortisol release), alpha-melanocyte stimulating hormone (which suppresses food intake in the brain and increases skin pigmentation in the body), beta-melanocyte stimulating hormone (which also affects food intake), and beta-endorphin. The mutation that I see most frequently in pre-opiomelanocortin changes the part of the protein that is 'cut' so that beta-endorphin is no longer made[92].

Patients with this variant tend to have very high anxiety and become easily distressed. Most patients lose their appetite during times of stress, and some also have problems with their gastrointestinal tract, like persistent nausea, vomiting, and diarrhea[93]. Most of the patients that I have seen would be classified as having 'atypical anorexia' because they are not sufficiently underweight to meet criteria for the traditional diagnosis of anorexia nervosa, and some studies have suggested that this variant can later increase the risk of obesity although the reports are not consistent[94] [95].

Gut-brain neuropeptides— Members of the gut-brain peptide group are largely expressed in the GI tract where they regulate digestion and absorption of food, and in the brain where they regulate behaviors related to eating. Neurotensin and its receptor, *neurotensin receptor 1,* are the two genes that we saw mutated most often in patients with anorexia in our original study in 2017[96]. Neurotensin is a member of the gut-brain neuropeptide group. Since the original study, I have found several additional patients with mutations in the neurotensin receptor 1, and they tend to be among my most difficult patients to treat.

The function of neurotensin itself is quite interesting and complicated. In the GI tract, neurotensin is released in response to the presence of food, particularly fat. Once it is released, neurotensin helps in the digestion and absorption of fat in several ways, including increasing blood flow to the intestines, and by increasing the release of digestive enzymes and bile to promote the absorption of fat. I have observed that most of my patients with mutations in neurotensin or its receptor tend to have difficulty with restoring weight and are often placed on very high calorie meal plans during treatment in order to gain weight. Lack of neurotensin could impair absorption of fat and be the cause of this difficulty with restoring weight.

The role of brain neurotensin in appetite is more complicated. Injecting rodents with neurotensin suppresses their appetite, and mice who do not have the neurotensin receptor 1 tend to overeat and gain weight when given high calorie food options. Both observations show that neurotensin is a <u>satiety</u> signal telling the brain to stop eating and telling the gut to digest and absorb the food that is present. However, mice without the neurotensin receptor 1 who are fed a low-calorie chow diet tend to eat less and become more physically active[97]. This effect of neurotensin is probably a result of acting on dopamine neurons in the brain reward system, because removing this subset of dopamine neurons from the brains of mice causes them to become hyperactive and lose weight[98]. These observations are more consistent with the behaviors of patients with anorexia who have a strong drive to exercise and decreased food intake. It is possible that both situations are true. Patients lacking neurotensin may in fact be predisposed to overeat high calorie foods and gain weight, but they are so afraid of developing obesity that they avoid these foods and instead eat blander, low-calorie options that lead them to eat less and over exercise.

Functions of Gut-Brain Neuropeptides

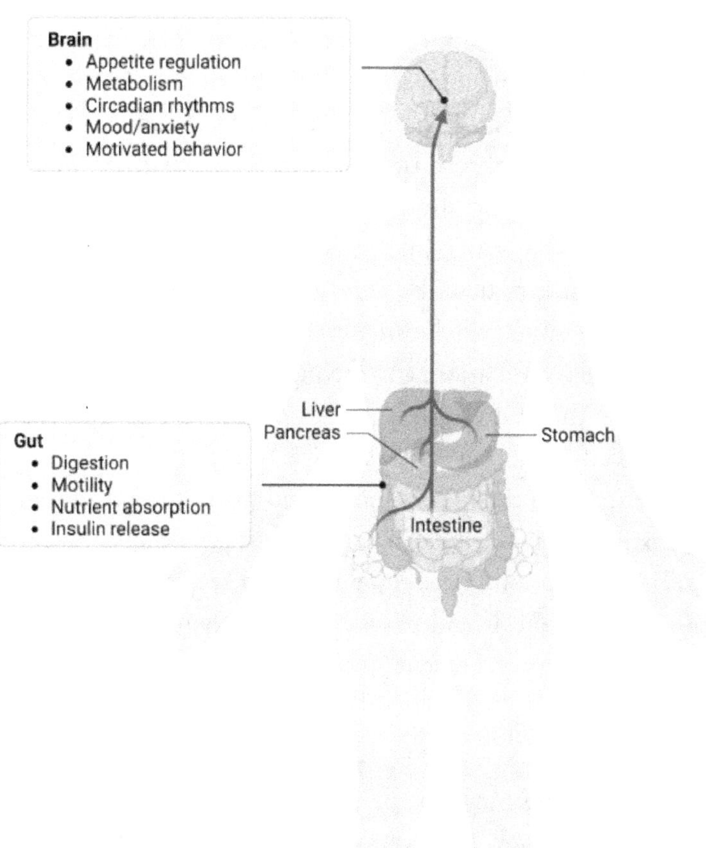

Gut-brain neuropeptides: There are several other members of the gut-brain peptide family that are also more likely to be mutated in patients with eating disorders, including genes *Prokineticin Receptor 1*, *Cholecystokinin Receptor A*, and *Vasoactive Intestinal Peptide Receptor 1*. These neuropeptides have many functions in the gastrointestinal tract after meals, including increasing motility (movement of food), blood flow, and secretion of digestive enzymes and bile. In the brain, these neuropeptides regulate many different processes, including <u>circadian rhythms</u>, blood flow, pain tolerance, and mood/anxiety.

Patients with mutations in these genes tend to be among my most volatile with severe cases of anorexia nervosa- binge/purge subtype. They often also have conditions like severe bipolar disorder and migraine headaches that complicate their treatment. These patients tend to be amongst my most severe in terms of self-induced vomiting and laxative abuse. This observation makes sense as these neuropeptides are important to the digestion of food, coordinating blood flow, motility, and release of water, bile, and digestive enzymes after a meal. Many of these patients describe very uncomfortable gastrointestinal symptoms after eating, including cramping, bloating, distention, heartburn, severe constipation, and feeling like the food is "just sitting there." I believe the desire to relieve this discomfort is what leads to the self-induced vomiting and laxative abuse in these patients. Unfortunately, at this time I have not found many good treatments to improve gastrointestinal tract function and reduce symptoms in these patients. The best option I have right now is to keep a regular schedule of consistent small meals and snacks, manage their mood symptoms and migraines, and try to prevent episodes of binging.

<u>Dopamine and Serotonin</u>

Dopamine and serotonin may be the two most famous of all the neurotransmitters. They are commonly associated with things like pleasure and happiness, because they are well-known targets of both psychiatric medications and drugs of abuse. For instance, drugs like cocaine and methamphetamine produce euphoria by greatly increasing levels of dopamine, which can also lead to addiction. Likewise certain medications used to treat major depression (like bupropion) and attention deficit hyperactivity disorder (like stimulants) also increase levels of dopamine, but to a much lesser degree than drugs of abuse. Much like dopamine, serotonin can also be the target of both medications (like fluoxetine) or drugs of abuse (LSD and ecstasy).

Dopamine and serotonin also regulate aspects of appetite and food intake. Too little dopamine causes an apathy syndrome including severe depression and a low desire to eat. Hormones that control appetite including leptin, ghrelin, and glucagon-like peptide 1 are thought to do so in part by affecting the activity of dopamine neurons[99][100]. Certain drugs, like cocaine and methamphetamine, can increase dopamine to unnaturally high levels, which also decreases appetite, while the stimulant medication lisdexamfetamine is approved by the Food and Drug Administration to treat binge-eating disorder. Serotonin affects food intake, primarily through the activity of the serotonin 2C receptor[101]. Activation of the serotonin 2C receptor suppresses appetite and was the target of two appetite suppressing drugs, fenfluramine and lorcaserin, that have since been removed from the market due to side effects.

So, it is probably not surprising that mutations in genes related to dopamine and serotonin functioning are sometimes seen in patients with eating disorders. I have found that patients with anorexia are more likely to have damaging mutations in genes involved in making a molecule called <u>tetrahydrobiopterin</u> (abbreviated as BH4). Tetrahydrobiopterin works primarily as a cofactor, which means that it helps other proteins do their job. One of its primary jobs is to help make the neurotransmitters dopamine and serotonin. The neurotransmitter norepinephrine is made from dopamine, so lack of tetrahydrobiopterin causes low levels of dopamine, norepinephrine, and dopamine— the three most common targets of antidepressant medications[102]. Another gene that I also frequently see mutated in patients with eating disorders is *TPH2*, which is involved in making serotonin (which is then turned into melatonin as well). These individuals have normal levels of dopamine and norepinephrine, but low levels of serotonin. Likewise, the gene *TH* makes a protein called Tyrosine Hydroxylase, which uses tetrahydrobiopterin to help make dopamine out of the amino acid tyrosine. Patients with mutations in the *TH* gene have normal levels of serotonin and melatonin, but low levels of dopamine and norepinephrine (see illustration on next page).

Synthesis of serotonin (left): The body makes the neurotransmitter serotonin from the amino acid tryptophan in a two step process. In step 1, tryptophan is turned into a molecule called 5-HTP by the protein tryptophan 5-hydroxylase (which is made from the *TPH1* gene in the body and the *TPH2* gene in the brain). In the step 2, 5-HTP is then converted into serotonin. Mutations in the *TPH1* or *TPH2* lead to decreased levels of serotonin in the brain or body. Patients with mutations in the *TPH* genes can benefit from the supplement 5-HTP.

Synthesis of dopamine and norepinephrine (right): The body makes the neurotransmitter dopamine from the amino acid tyrosine. In step 1, tyrosine is turned into a molecule called DOPA by the protein tyrosine hydroxylase (which is made from the *TH* gene). DOPA is then converted into dopamine in step 2. The neurotransmitter norepinephrine is then made from dopamine by the protein dopamine β-hydroxylase.

Both tryptophan 5-hydroxylase and tyrosine hydroxylase require the cofactor tetrahydrobiopterin (shown as BH4 in the middle). Patients with mutations in genes involved in making BH4 have low levels of serotonin, dopamine, and norepinephrine.

<u>Circadian Rhythms</u>

Most people are aware that our behaviors are linked to a day/night cycle. While sleep is the most obvious example of a behavior linked to the day/night cycle, there are numerous processes that are more likely to occur at a specific time of day. Hunger, body temperature, glucose storage, and cardiovascular functioning are all optimized to function during the daytime, while sleep, urine concentration, glucose release, and restorative processes preferentially occur at night.

Any bodily activity that fluctuates on a 24-hour cycle is called a <u>circadian rhythm</u>[103]. What many people might not be aware of, though, is that circadian rhythms are hardwired into the DNA. There are a set of genes whose primary function is to mark the length of the day and to coordinate bodily activities with your body's clock to optimize functioning. Because many organisms on the planet experience day/night cycles, circadian rhythms are found all throughout both the plant and animal kingdoms, which has allowed for the discovery of the genes that regulate this process.

The core circadian clock is composed of a series of proteins that are made from genes with names like *CLOCK, BMAL1, NR1D1, PERIOD,* and *CRYPTOCHROME.* The proteins CLOCK, BMAL1, and REV-ERB (which is the name of the protein that is made from the *NR1D1* gene) are all <u>transcription factors</u>, which means that they are proteins that control the expression of other genes. Transcription factors are very important in the body because they coordinate entire biological processes. You can think of transcription factors sort of like a party planner. When you hire a party planner, they will help reserve a location, plan the decorations, order the food, hire the entertainment, and send out the invitations. The party planner makes sure that you have all the things you need for a party to take place. Transcription factors act much like party planners to make sure you have all the proteins your cells need in order to complete a certain task. In fact, the very first gene mutation I found that increases the risk of developing anorexia was in a transcription factor called ESRRA[104], which increases the levels of proteins involved in making <u>mitochondria</u> and in burning fatty acids or amino acids. Other famous transcription factors include the estrogen and testosterone receptors, which control genes involved in sexual development, and the vitamin D receptor, which controls genes involved in calcium and phosphorus levels in the body.

CLOCK and BMAL1 are transcription factors that control circadian rhythms by increasing the production of proteins that are necessary during the day and decreasing the amount of those proteins at night. Likewise, CLOCK and BMAL1 also increase the production of proteins that your body uses at night and then decrease those proteins during the day. A good example of this is a hormone called vasopressin (antidiuretic hormone). Vasopressin tells your kidneys to concentrate your urine so that you make less volume of it. CLOCK and BMAL increase the levels of vasopressin, but only at night so that you don't have to get up multiple times throughout the night to go to the bathroom (that is why your urine in the morning can be dark yellow)[105]. During the daytime, CLOCK and BMAL1 keep vasopressin levels low so that your kidneys make larger amounts of urine. But this is just one example. In total, up to 10% of our genes may cycle up and down during the day[106].

This internal clock can run on its own, at least for a short period of time. If you place a person or animal in complete darkness, vasopressin levels will still rise and fall on a nearly 24-hour cycle for several days. The circadian cycle can also be fine-tuned to better line up with daily activities in a person's life. For instance, the circadian clock needs to reset if you are flying to a new time zone or switching to a job where you work an overnight shift. The body can reset your circadian clock by using signals from the outside world like daylight (specifically blue light), temperature, physical activity, and the availability of food, which are called zeitgebers from the German meaning 'time givers[107]'. Zeitgebers send signals to neurons in the brain to either shorten or lengthen the length of each circadian cycle a little bit every day until the new circadian rhythm lines up again with the outside world.

The Circadian Clock

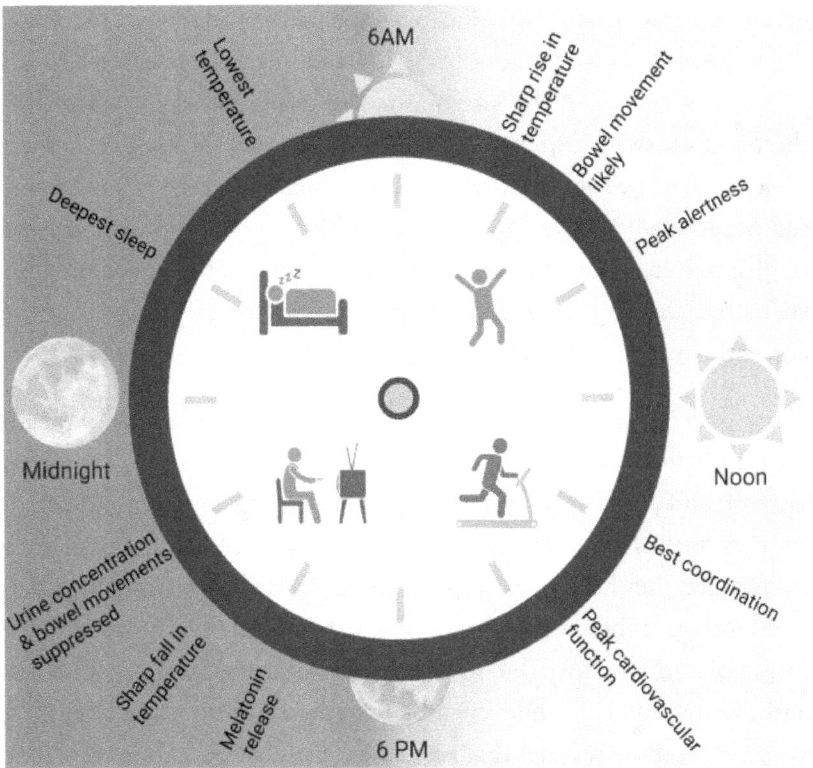

Circadian rhythms are powerful regulators of behavior, as anyone with young children has experienced when the family must adapt to daylight savings time. Even shifts in timing as small as one hour can greatly affect things like sleep, hunger, alertness, and concentration. It therefore probably comes as no surprise that mutations in the genes of the circadian clock can have profound effects on the behavior as well. In eating disorder patients, I frequently see mutations in several circadian rhythm genes, including *CLOCK*, *PERIOD*, and *CRYPTOCHROME*. Patients with circadian disruptions have much different presentations than other patients with eating disorders.

First, they tend to have much more disrupted sleep patterns, with most of my patients displaying a delayed sleep phase, that is, they prefer to go to bed much later than most people. In one extreme case, I had a school-aged patient whose preferred time to go to sleep is around 5 AM and get up in the afternoon. The change in sleep schedule is then coupled with extreme changes in meal patterns as well. If these patients go to bed at their preferred time, then they sleep right through the traditional times for breakfast and lunch. If they get up at a more traditional time like 6 or 7 AM for school or work, then they are often very tired and have little appetite (imagine trying to get up at 1 AM and eating your breakfast).

These patients are not without an appetite though. They will typically eat very little breakfast or lunch and then be very hungry after school or work and either snack excessively or have a large dinner followed by another 'meal' later in the evening around midnight. Patients will often be told that they have an eating disorder because they 'restrict' breakfast and lunch and then 'binge' at night, but I think that in most cases the eating disturbances are due to the chronic effects of sleep deprivation and misalignment of their circadian rhythms. These patients tend to struggle in school settings that require early morning attendance but do very well later in life where they tend to gravitate to jobs that are later in the evening, like live entertainment, nursing, or airline pilots that fly the red eye (one bonus is that many of these jobs tend to be higher paying as well because of the less desirable times).

One special subset of patients with circadian rhythm disruptions are the so-called 'short sleepers.' While most adults prefer 7 to 10 hours of sleep, these individuals only need 4 to 5 hours per night. They also tend to be very positive, productive, and accomplished. Because of these traits, short sleepers tend to be very successful and are over-represented in positions of leadership. I have personally had patients who were university professors, scientists, and corporate executives. While they tend to be very resilient, they have a very characteristic response to times of extreme stress. At first, they will lose their appetite and begin to sleep less. This period is often associated with an increase in physical activity as well. Eventually, as their sleep drops to 1 to 3 hours per night and they lose a significant amount of weight, their eating will switch, and they will begin binging on extremely large amounts of carbohydrates[108]. At this point, the patient will often present for eating disorder treatment with a diagnosis of either anorexia nervosa-binge/purge subtype (if they are underweight), bulimia nervosa-non-purging subtype (if they compulsively exercise), or binge eating disorder (if neither is present).

Recognizing the presence of a circadian rhythm disruption is critical because it greatly changes the type of treatment the patient needs. Most of the time, simply talking to a patient about what a typical day is like for them will be enough to suspect the presence of a circadian rhythm disorder. From there, circadian rhythms can also be easily measured by using wearable devices to monitor factors such as physical activity, sleep patterns, or body temperature. Once several days' worth of monitoring has been collected, the data can then be lined up to create a chart showing the length and phase of each patient's natural rhythm. I refer to this preferred phase as the patient's 'chronotype.'

After identifying the chronotype of the patient, the next step is to create a treatment plan that reinforces this rhythm, which I call <u>Circadian Entrainment Therapy</u>. My approach is to schedule strong zeitgebers throughout the day to strengthen the clock. A typical schedule would include going to bed at the same time every night, using a sunlight simulating alarm clock if needed to help with waking up in the morning, physical activity or a hot shower in the morning to help increase body temperature, having meals and medications around the same time every day, taking a small dose of melatonin around sunset, blue light filters after sunset, and sleeping in a cool, dark room. For patients who are short sleepers, I try to get them back to sleeping closer to 5 to 6 hours if possible and using sleep medications when they notice that they are starting to slip back into sleeping shorter and shorter lengths of time each night.

Endocannabinoids

The endocannabinoid system is similar in many ways to the opioid system. Most people are more familiar with the exogenous cannabinoids that are used as medications or as recreational drugs, like marijuana. Like the opioid system, the body also makes its own endocannabinoids and has its own cannabinoid receptors. One major difference is that while the receptors for cannabinoids are proteins that are made from genes (called *CNR1* and *CNR2*), the endocannabinoid neurotransmitters are not proteins made from a gene but, rather, are made from lipids after a neuron is stimulated by a neurotransmitter. The primary endocannabinoids are anandamide and 2-arachidonoylglycerol, and they also have one other important difference compared to other neurotransmitters. Instead of moving from the firing neuron to the target neuron, endocannabinoids move in the reverse direction of other neurotransmitters: they are released by the target neuron and inhibit the firing of the original neuron, decreasing the release of other neurotransmitters (see illustration on next page). You can think of it as a sort of brake system. A neuron will release a molecule like glutamate which will then bind to another neuron and cause it to fire. This firing of the neuron also causes the production and release of endocannabinoids like anandamide and 2-arachidonoylglycerol, which then move backwards to turn off the further release of glutamate from the original neuron. Anandamide and 2-arachidonoylglycerol are then broken down by the action of certain enzymes called Fatty Acid Amide Hydrolases (which are made from the genes *FAAH1* and *FAAH2*) and the whole cycle can begin again with the firing of the original neuron.

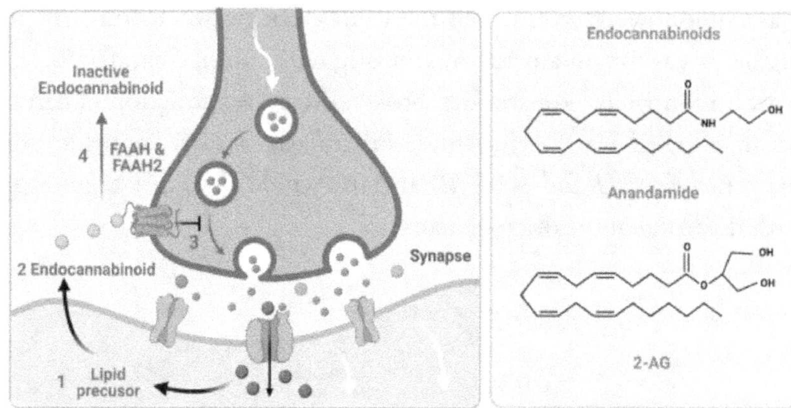

The endocannabinoid system: Endocannabinoids work in the 'opposite' direction as most traditional neurotransmitters. 1. They are released after after a neuron has been activated neuron and then 2. move backward and bind to receptors on the original neuron called the cannabinoid receptor. 3. Cannabinoid receptors can now inhibit neurotransmitter release acting like a 'brake' to shut off the first neuron. 4. Proteins like FAAH and FAAH2 breakdown the endocannabinoids allowing the top neuron to release neurotransmitters again (left).

Examples of different types of endocannabinoids (right).

The Cannabinoid Receptor 1 is expressed widely throughout the body, especially in the brain, but the Cannabinoid Receptor 2 is primarily located in the brain and immune system. The endocannabinoid system regulates a broad array of functions in the brain, including alertness, pain, memory, motor coordination, appetite, and sexual functioning. In the body, endocannabinoids affect things like metabolism in the liver, adipose tissues, and muscles, as well as inflammation caused by the immune system. Exogenous (or external) activation of the cannabinoid system by consumption of marijuana has several effects, including sedation, euphoria, memory impairment, and appetite stimulation. A drug that blocks the action of the cannabinoid receptor 1, called rimonabant, was briefly approved as a weight loss medication in some countries, but it was removed worldwide in 2008 because it caused psychiatric side effects, including increased risk of anxiety, depression, and suicidal thoughts[109].

Within the patients that I treat, I have most often seen mutations in *FAAH* and *FAAH2* genes in patients with restrictive eating patterns, and in the *Cannabinoid Receptor 2* gene in patients with binge-eating. FAAH and FAAH2 are involved in breaking down endocannabinoids, so it would be predicted that individuals with these mutations would have higher levels of endocannabinoids. This may at first seem counterintuitive because cannabinoid receptor signaling is typically associated with appetite stimulation. One possible explanation is that having high levels of cannabinoid signaling your entire life leads the system to become overwhelmed. Indeed, we are starting to see something like this in patients who smoke large amounts of high potency marijuana. Some of these patients will develop a disorder called <u>cannabinoid hyperemesis syndrome</u>[110], which is characterized by persistent nausea, lack of appetite, weight loss, and abdominal pain. In severe cases, patients may have uncontrollable vomiting that requires hospitalization. It is plausible, then, that some patients with mutations in *FAAH* and *FAAH2* have a milder, but chronic form of this illness due to genetic mutations that persistently elevate endocannabinoid levels.

The role of Cannabinoid Receptor 2 in binge eating behaviors is more straightforward. Activation of Cannabinoid Receptor 2 tends to suppress appetite in mice[111], and mice that lack Cannabinoid Receptor 2 have higher food intake and develop obesity[112]. These findings suggest that unlike Cannabinoid Receptor 1, which stimulates appetite, Cannabinoid Receptor 2 inhibits food intake and may act as a counterbalance to the appetite stimulating effects of substances like marijuana. Patients with damaging mutations in Cannabinoid Receptor 2 lose this counterbalance and shift more toward the appetite stimulating effects of Cannabinoid Receptor 1.

<u>Vitamin D</u>

<u>Vitamin D</u> deficiency has become one of the trendy areas of medicine recently, with Vitamin D supplementation being touted to help improve mood, weight loss, and prevent a wide variety of diseases, including heart disease, COVID-19, and autoimmune disorders[113]. Within the field of eating disorders, vitamin D supplementation is used to help prevent osteoporosis, especially in patients with anorexia who may be at higher risk of developing osteoporosis due to low estrogen levels that come from being underweight.

While I was vaguely aware of Vitamin D, it was certainly not something I ever considered as a contributing factor to the risk of getting an eating disorder until I started doing whole exome sequencing. I have now identified several patients with eating disorders who have mutations in the *Klotho* and *Cytochrome P450 family 24 subfamily A member 1 (CYP24A1)* genes. The proteins made from these two genes play a critical role in controlling the levels of vitamin D, calcium, and phosphorus in the body.

To better understand how these mutations might contribute to an eating disorder, it would first be helpful to review how they work. Vitamin D can be made either from the skin in response to sunlight or taken in from foods that you eat. This form of vitamin D is then turned into a molecule called 25-hydroxy-vitamin D by the liver and then, finally, it is changed into its active form called 1,25-dihydroxy-vitamin D (also called calcitriol). In its active form, 1,25-dihydroxy-vitamin D is very important for maintaining the proper levels of the electrolytes calcium and phosphorus. It does this in several ways. First, 1,25-dihydroxy-vitamin D can increase the absorption of calcium and phosphorus from your food in your intestines. Second, it can reabsorb calcium from the kidney so that it is not lost in the urine. Finally, it can break down bone and release calcium and phosphorus if needed to maintain blood levels

Calcium is important for many functions in the body, including bone formation and conduction of electrical impulses in the neurons and heart. Phosphorus is a key component of bone as well and is also part of ATP— the molecule I mentioned earlier that is the primary source of energy used by the cells in your body. Elevated levels of calcium and phosphorus can lead to the formation of small mineral deposits in the blood vessels called calcifications, which can cause cardiovascular disease and accelerate the aging process.

Since maintaining proper levels of calcium and phosphorus is critical for health, vitamin D levels are also tightly controlled by the body. The active form of vitamin D is primarily broken down by the protein CYP24A1, which turns it into an inactive molecule called calcitroic acid. Active vitamin D has one other important way that it regulates itself— by increasing the amount of Klotho. Klotho, along with a hormone called FGF23, helps maintain vitamin D levels by increasing its breakdown of CYP24A1 and by decreasing the production of new active Vitamin D from its precursor 25-hydroxy-vitamin D in the liver. In this way, it helps maintain levels of vitamin D within a very tight range.

Mutations that damage the functioning of CYP24A1 or Klotho proteins can lead to elevated levels of vitamin D and potentially high levels of calcium and phosphorus, as well. The symptoms of vitamin D toxicity include loss of appetite, fatigue, gastrointestinal complaints like nausea and constipation, and depressed mood or brain fog. All these symptoms can worsen the symptoms of major depression and eating disorders. One other observation that I have made is that many of my eating disorder patients with mutations in *CYP24A1* or *Klotho* also have a neurological disorder, like multiple sclerosis or epilepsy. It is not clear that these are directly related, but there have been links observed between vitamin D and these disorders before[114],[115].

I would like to make one more observation about vitamin D before moving on. Medical providers typically measure levels of 25-hydroxy-vitamin D and not the active form 1,25-dihydroxy-vitamin D. In most cases, this does not make a difference because low levels of 25-hydroxy-vitamin D also indicate low levels of 1,25-dihydroxy-vitamin D. This correlation falls apart, though, in patients with mutations in *CYP24A1* or *Klotho*. As you may recall, Klotho and FGF23 go to the kidney and block it from changing 25-hydroxy-vitamin D into active 1,25-dihydroxy-vitamin D. Without this brake on the system, most of the 25-hydroxy-vitamin D is used up and the levels appear to be very low even though levels of the active 1,25-dihydroxy-Vitamin D are normal or high. This matters because I have found several instances where well-meaning medical providers find that a patient has low levels of 25-hydroxy-Vitamin D and start giving them large doses of vitamin D to get their levels into the normal range, but inadvertently cause vitamin D toxicity.

<u>Sleep Disorders</u>

Sleep and food intake are closely linked. As we discussed earlier, both sleep and appetite are controlled by the circadian clock, but other connections exist as well. Transitions between being awake and being asleep are controlled by a small set of neurons in the brain that make a peptide neurotransmitter called orexin. Orexin promotes being awake, and orexin neurons are active during the day and then turn off at night, allowing sleep to occur. Destruction of orexin-containing neurons by the immune system causes the disease narcolepsy, in which patients have unpredictable bouts of sleep.

Being awake at the right time is obviously very important for survival, though so orexin neurons are controlled by many other things besides whether it is night or day outside. One of the primary regulators of orexin activity is the presence of glucose. Glucose inhibits the activity of orexin neurons[116] while low glucose levels potently activate orexin neurons[117]. This makes logical sense, as having low blood sugar levels is a time when you need to be awake and forging for food, while taking a nap after a meal is also very common.

So, if food intake regulates sleep, could the opposite also be true? Could disrupted sleep affect your appetite? I recently identified a subgroup of patients with a mutation in the gene *KCNQ2*. The protein product of this gene is an ion channel that allows for the passage of positively charged potassium molecules to control the electrical excitability of orexin neurons. Put differently, it controls how easy or how hard it is to make an orexin neuron fire[118]. When KCNQ2 protein levels are low, it makes orexin neurons more easily excited, which leads to frequent awakening at night.

I have found that patients with mutations in the KCNQ2 gene often wake up frequently throughout the night, sometimes as many as 10 times per night, and have trouble going back to sleep. Some of the patients describe getting up in the middle of the night during these times and getting something to eat, which helps them go back to sleep. They are sometimes diagnosed with night eating syndrome (which is listed as one of the disorders under other specified eating and feeding disorders or OSFED). Putting these findings together now, the cause for their night eating becomes clearer. Mutations in KCNQ2 lead to overactive orexin neurons, which causes people to wake up in the middle of the night and not be able to go back to sleep. Over time, they learn that eating something will increase their glucose levels which could potentially inhibit orexin neurons and allow them to go back to sleep. The key to treating these patients is to treat the underlying sleep disorder by using sleep medications that block the action of orexin, which allows them to sleep through the night and prevents the night eating.

In this chapter and the previous one, I described many different genetic mutations I and others have uncovered that seem to drive eating disorders and related diseases and syndromes. Notably, this list of genetic mechanisms remains incomplete, and many more genetic and environmental causes of these diseases remain to be found. The key takeaway from these observations, though, is that understanding the genetic causes of an individual patient's symptoms can help determine the most effective methods of treatment and may even lead to new treatment methods that could help many other patients. In the next chapter, I will lay out my vision for doing exactly this.

Chapter 9: The Promise and Peril of Repurposing Drugs

Once you find a biological pathway that is affected in a disorder like major depression or anorexia, the next major question is what can you do about it? With a few exceptions, most pathways that I have found to have damaging genetic mutations are not treated with traditional psychiatric medications. In this chapter, I will review how we can use our newfound knowledge of the underlying causes of psychiatric disorders to repurpose medications that are already clinically available for use.

So how do you go about trying to find a treatment for the only person in the world with a certain mutation? Let's do a thought experiment and imagine what the ideal new treatment for a psychiatric condition would be from a patient's point of view. Ideally a treatment would have the following features[119]:

1. It would greatly improve symptoms.
2. It would be well tolerated with good safety data and minimal side effects.
3. It would be inexpensive and easy to take or easy to administer.

New treatments in psychiatry rarely have all three of these features. Most new medications that come to market are so-called 'me-too' drugs because they are slightly changed versions of older medications that are already on the market. Pharmaceutical companies can take these older medications and modify them enough for a new patent to be awarded. This newer medication can then be taken through the FDA approval process by doing a <u>randomized controlled trial</u> against a placebo medication. Because this new 'me-too' medication is not required to be compared head-to-head against the older medications, we do not know if it works any better than generic alternatives that are already available. These new medications are not any less expensive though, even if they are just modified versions of older medications.

Most generic medications cost 80-85% less than medications still on patent[120].

One class of medications that do fit all three of the criteria above are so-called 'repurposed' medications. Repurposed medications are drugs that have already been FDA approved from another condition (the 'on-label' use) but can legally be prescribed for 'off-label' use of another condition if a doctor thinks that the medication might be helpful and the patient consents to treatment. Repurposed medications tend to excel in criteria #2, they have often been prescribed for decades, which means that relatively cheap generic versions are available. They also fulfill criteria #3, having years of safety data available for large numbers of patients.

The more difficult part is satisfying criteria #1— identifying new uses for old medications. Medication trials are expensive, especially the gold-standard randomized controlled trial. Small trials can cost hundreds of thousands of dollars, and large trials can run into the tens of millions[121]. Pharmaceutical companies are willing to pay this cost for new medications because of their ability to charge high prices during the life of the patent, but there is no such incentive for studies of repurposed medications. Without a profit motive to encourage private industry to conduct a research study, the only other group of researchers able to do repurposing studies are scientists at major research universities and academic medical centers. In theory, it is possible to see if a repurposed medication is effective for treating a different condition by writing a grant that would cover the cost of studying an older medication for a new purpose. These types of grants are much smaller though, because they usually come from either the National Institute of Health or patient advocacy groups, which have less resources. As a result, the size of the trials and number of patients tested tends to be smaller.

Once a repurposed medication is found to have a new use, there is a second problem of marketing that use to doctors and patients. Pharmaceutical companies run sophisticated marketing campaigns with the ability to reach millions of patients and thousands of doctors through TV commercials, internet ads, and sales representatives. Within a few days of a new medication becoming available to be prescribed, I will have a sales representative from a pharmaceutical company knock on my office door to give me information on how to prescribe their drug. Pharmaceutical companies can also increase awareness of their new medication by giving money to cover the cost of scientific meetings, hiring speakers to give presentations on their behalf, and paying for awareness programs for the conditions that their medications are used to treat. This practice is especially common if a new medication is approved for a condition that did not previously have a treatment.

A good example of this occurred when the medication Vyvanse got an FDA approval to treat binge eating disorder in 2015. Binge eating disorder only became an official Diagnostic and Statistical Manual Diagnosis in 2013 and, prior to Vyvanse, there were no FDA approved medications to treat binge eating disorder. In order to make both the general public and doctors aware that episodes of binge eating could now be diagnosed as an illness, Shire, the company that makes Vyvanse, launched a marketing campaign that included hiring a celebrity spokesperson, creating a website with information on binge eating disorder, and partnering with patient advocacy groups[122]. Shire was able to do this because once there is an FDA-approved indication for a medication, insurance companies must cover the cost. Because Vyvanse was also the first FDA-approved medication for binge eating disorder, it also meant there was no generic competition (if there are generic and non-generic medications for an illness, insurance companies will often require that you try the generic option first before they will pay for the more expensive brand-name medication). This financial incentive justified the cost of these programs to raise awareness about the existence of binge eating disorder as a diagnosis.

In the case of repurposed medications, there is no financial incentive to promote a new use for an old medication. So, even if a researcher at a university can get funding and complete the study, it can be very difficult to get the broader medical field to start using the new treatment. A prime example of this is the use of prazosin for post-traumatic stress disorder (PTSD)-related nightmares. Prazosin is an older blood pressure medication that is primarily used now to treat swelling of the prostate that blocks urine flow in older men[123]. In 2000, a group of researchers working at the Veterans Affairs Hospital first reported that prazosin reduces nightmares that occur in patients with post-traumatic stress disorder[124]. Prazosin can lower blood pressure but is otherwise generally well-tolerated and very inexpensive (less than $10 per month as of this writing). Analysis of multiple studies on prazosin for trauma-related nightmares has found that it is safe and effective in adults[125] and adolescents[126]. I have not treated patients in a Veterans Affairs Hospital since 2007, but my understanding is that its use for military trauma-related nightmares is well known in that system. Use of prazosin for nightmares related to civilian post-traumatic stress disorder is less known, however. Less than half of my patients with trauma-related nightmares who have received treatment before are offered prazosin by another medical provider before I see them.

Repurposed drugs have one other major advantage— they are available immediately. While some patients do find it helpful to know about mutations that might be contributing to their illness, most patients just want to feel better. So, identifying a potential pathway to treat is of little value to someone if they must wait years or decades for a new drug to be developed.

<u>The Example of Ketamine</u>

Perhaps the single best case of a repurposed medication in the field of psychiatry is the use of ketamine for major depression. The story of ketamine highlights both the immense potential and the immense barriers to repurposing medications.

Ketamine was first used clinically as an <u>anesthetic</u>[127] in the 1960s and came to be used widely in combat settings because it was more stable and easier to administer than other anesthetics at the time[128]. Over the decades, it gradually fell out of favor as other medications with fewer <u>psychoactive</u> side effects became available, that is, until 2006, when researchers at the National Institute of Mental Health found that giving lower doses of ketamine intravenously produced a rapid antidepressant effect[129].

This finding was considered a major breakthrough at the time because it was the first medication that treated depression in a different way to become available in decades. The first antidepressant was discovered by accident when a medication used to treat tuberculosis, called iproniazid, was also found to have antidepressant effects[130]. Scientists eventually determined that iproniazid increases levels of three neurotransmitters in the brain— dopamine, serotonin, and norepinephrine. Every antidepressant that followed iproniazid was based upon boosting levels of one or more of these neurotransmitters until ketamine was identified in 2006. Ketamine works by targeting a different neurotransmitter in the brain called glutamate. Glutamate is the opposite of the inhibitory neurotransmitter GABA that we discussed earlier, because glutamate causes neurons to fire instead of inhibiting their firing.

Because ketamine works differently, it distinguished itself from other antidepressants available at the time. It tends to work quickly, within hours or days instead of months or years, and worked for some individuals for whom traditional antidepressants that target dopamine, serotonin, and norepinephrine did not work. There is also evidence that ketamine reduces suicidal thinking, a major concern for which there are limited treatments available[131].

The story of what happens next with ketamine highlights the barriers to using old medications for new purposes. Ketamine itself costs only a few dollars. So, the primary cost in giving patients ketamine is paying for someone to administer the intravenous infusions and monitor the patients afterwards. The first problem, though, is that ketamine is not FDA-approved to treat major depression, so while it is legal to prescribe it for 'off-label' use, insurance companies are not required to pay for it. There are ketamine infusion clinics that have popped up mostly around major urban areas, but these clinics typically require patients to pay several hundred dollars out of pocket per infusion, which limits the number of people who can get the treatments. Because the patent had expired on ketamine, there was no financial incentive for a pharmaceutical company to conduct a large randomized controlled trial and go through the FDA-approval process to get ketamine approved to treat major depression.

Pharmaceutical companies do have one strategy, though, for situations like this where a patent has expired for an older medication. Many molecules, including ketamine, exist in two forms as mirror images of each other (a concept known as chirality). You can think of it like a right and left hand. Each hand has a thumb, fore finger, middle finger, ring finger, and pinky on each hand, but in the opposite orientation. You would not be able to put the right hand in a left glove and vice versa. Likewise, ketamine exists as a mixture of two mirror images called esketamine and arketamine[132]. Unlike ketamine, esketamine and arketamine can be patented even though ketamine is just a mixture of the two. There are several famous medications that have used this approach. The acid blocking medication Nexium (esomeprazole) is just one of the two mirror images of an older medication Prilosec (omeprazole). Likewise, the antidepressant Lexapro (escitalopram) is just half of the older antidepressant Celexa (citalopram) with a new patent and a better marketing campaign.

The pharmaceutical company Johnson and Johnson took advantage of this loophole and got esketamine approved by the FDA for use as a rapidly acting antidepressant in 2019. Interestingly, Johnson and Johnson decided to drop intravenous infusions in favor of using a nasal spray to deliver the medication instead. I am not sure why they decided to take this approach, but they may have felt that creating a network of infusion centers to do intravenous infusions was too difficult or would limit the number of people who could get the medication. They also may have worried that once insurance companies were forced to pay for esketamine plus the intravenous infusions, they would eventually just agree to pay for infusions of the cheaper generic ketamine instead. In any event, esketamine as a nasal spray can now be administered at psychiatry clinics around the country with special monitoring.

There is just one problem with intranasal esketamine, though: early reports suggest that intravenous ketamine appears to work better than intranasal esketamine[133]. I have witnessed similar outcomes in my own patients who received intravenous ketamine and had better results than patients receiving intranasal treatments. Intranasal esketamine also costs more money— between $590-885 per dose[134]. The initial phase of treatment requires two doses per week for one month, resulting in a total cost of $4,720 to $6,785 to start the treatment, with future treatments given either once a week or once every two weeks.

Of course, few people pay this price themselves. Because esketamine is FDA-approved, it must be covered by insurance, but that does not stop the insurance companies from putting up administrative hurdles to cross in order to get the cost of the treatment covered.

So, the final result of the initial 2006 finding that intravenous ketamine is effective as a rapidly acting antidepressant is that we have ended up with intranasal esketamine, which may be less effective and more expensive. It does create enormous profits, though, for pharmaceutical companies, doctor's offices, researchers, and marketers. In the end, I fear that the only way to get broad adoption of a new treatment is for all the parties involved to get a slice of the profits.

How Whole Exome Sequencing Can Help Medication Repurposing

One of the most surprising personally satisfying things I have discovered from using whole exome sequencing is how often a genetic finding leads to a simple, straightforward treatment that we would not have considered without doing the testing. Many of these treatments involve the use of repurposed medications, but at other times, they involve vitamins or supplements that are widely available, inexpensive, and have good safety data available (at least in the fields of eating disorders and depression). My hope is that precision medicine techniques will encourage psychiatrists to start seeking out new treatments, especially when the traditional options have not worked. In the next section, I will explore some examples of treatments that I have identified for my patients based upon whole exome sequencing.

Rapamycin—In chapter 8, I presented my view that anorexia nervosa is the result of errors in metabolism that trigger activation of the mTOR pathway. The logical question that arises from this idea is whether a medication that inhibits the activity of mTOR could be used to decrease the symptoms of anorexia. Medications that inhibit mTOR, like rapamycin, already exist and have been FDA-approved to prevent the immune system from attacking organ transplants[135]. While rapamycin and related medications are typically used daily at high doses in order to suppress the immune system after an organ transplant, researchers are now studying medications that inhibit mTOR to see if they can be used at lower doses or less frequently to treat a variety of conditions, including certain types of cancer[136], and certain forms of seizures[137], and even preventing aging[138]. The use of mTOR inhibitors has touched psychiatry as well. A group of researchers found that giving patients an mTOR inhibitor prior to receiving an infusion of ketamine prolonged the antidepressant effects of the ketamine[139], suggesting that mTOR signaling may be involved in antidepressant responses as well.

Medications that inhibit mTOR, like rapamycin could be a potential new treatment for certain cases of anorexia and target the underlying eating disorder thoughts and feelings. Because mTOR signaling has broad effects throughout the body, though, it does have several side effects, including anemia, elevated cholesterol, mouth ulcers, and problems with blood clotting[140]. So, it might be necessary to use rapamycin as a starting point to develop more specific medications for patients with anorexia that have fewer side effects. Another possibility is that rapamycin could be combined with other medications to decrease the amount of the drug that is needed to treat anorexia nervosa. One possibility is to combine rapamycin with ketamine. We discussed above how giving rapamycin before an infusion of ketamine prolongs the antidepressant effects of the ketamine infusion. Early studies have suggested that ketamine may benefit patients with anorexia[141][142][143] ,as well. Thus, it may be possible to use limited doses of rapamycin to enhance the effects of ketamine. The result would be the utilization of lower amounts of both drugs, which would cost less and hopefully have fewer side effects.

Vitamins and supplements— One of the very first things that jumped out to me when I started looking at genetic mutations in patients with anorexia nervosa was the number of mutations in genes related to vitamins and cofactors involved in metabolism. As we discussed earlier in chapter 8, your body's metabolism involves a set of very complex chemical reactions that are needed to turn the food that you eat into energy for your body to use. These chemical reactions require several vitamins and cofactors in order to break down carbohydrates, proteins, and fats into smaller molecules called acetyl-CoA that your <u>mitochondria</u> can use to make energy.

Essential vitamins are molecules that your body must get from food because it cannot make them on its own. The vitamins most often affected in patients with anorexia include several members of the <u>vitamin B complex:</u> thiamine (B1), niacin (B3), pantothenic acid (B5), pyridoxine (B6), biotin (B7), folate (B9) and cobalamin (B12). Cofactors are molecules that your body can either make on its own or that you can get in your diet. There are several genes required to make cofactors necessary for metabolism that are more likely to be mutated in patients with anorexia, including <u>carnitine</u>, <u>Co-Q10</u>, and <u>lipoic acid</u>.

It's important to note that regardless of where they come from, all these vitamins and cofactors require certain proteins (which are made by instructions from the genes in your DNA) for your body to use them. For example, there are certain proteins that are involved in helping your intestines absorb B1 and B12 from your diet and transport them into your cells for use. Once these vitamins are in your body, many of them require additional chemical reactions before your cells can use them. These chemical reactions are carried out by enzymes (which again are proteins made from the genes in your DNA). Examples of this include the conversion of folate into L-methylfolate, the conversion of thiamine into thiamine pyrophosphate, and the conversion of pantothenic acid into coenzyme A. Similarly, the body has certain enzymes involved in making L-carnitine, Co-Q10, and lipoic acid. These vitamins and cofactors are used extensively in metabolism. For instance, the enzymes that break down branched chain amino acids alone use vitamins B1, B3, B5, B6, B8, and B12 as well as carnitine and lipoic acid. My theory is that deficiencies in these vitamins and cofactors impair metabolism and lead to a buildup of fatty acids and amino acids that activates mTOR, leading to aversion to food and further restriction.

While some of the mutations in the genes related to vitamins and cofactors are difficult to overcome, most cases can be treated either by giving extra amounts of the vitamin or cofactor, or by giving a version of the vitamin or cofactor that is easier for the body to absorb, such as an injection into muscle, or a tablet that dissolves under the tongue.

Tetrahydrobiopterin— As I mentioned before, I have several patients with mutations in the genes involved in making the cofactor tetrahydrobiopterin, which is needed to make dopamine and serotonin. These patients tend to have severe anhedonia (inability to experience pleasure), including a very low desire to eat. They also tend to have severe symptoms of depression and do not respond well to traditional antidepressants. I would love to treat these patients with tetrahydrobiopterin, but right now, the only medical use of tetrahydrobiopterin is to treat certain types of phenylketonuria (a rare disease in which the body is unable to break down the amino acid phenylalanine) and it costs over $100,000 per year.

There are other options to help these patients though. L-dopa is a medication used to treat Parkinson's disease. L-dopa can be taken up by neurons and turned into dopamine without the need for tetrahydrobiopterin. L-dopa could normalize low levels of dopamine, although the long-term use of L-dopa is associated with side effects like unwanted muscle movements, which could make the risks not worth any potential benefits. Many of my patients with tetrahydrobiopterin deficiency also have a disorder called restless leg syndrome, in which patients often have an uncomfortable urge to move their legs, oftentimes causing them to wake up while sleeping. There is a group of medications used to treat restless leg syndrome that act like dopamine in the brain. I have used medications in this class, like pramipexole and ropinirole, to treat patients with mutations in the tetrahydrobiopterin gene and it seems to help symptoms of major depression and sleep as well. Finally, the supplement 5-HTP is a precursor to serotonin that does not need the presence of tetrahydrobiopterin. 5-HTP is widely available and can be given to patients with either mutations in the tetrahydrobiopterin pathway or the *THP2* gene to help normalize serotonin levels.

GLP-1 agonists— Earlier in the book, I reported that in 2017 we identified that mutations in the gene glucagon-like peptide 1 (GLP-1) were seen in patients with bulimia nervosa. GLP-1 is a <u>satiety</u> factor that helps people feel full and stop eating during a meal, so we hypothesized that this lack of satiety contributes to the binge eating behaviors in patients with bulimia. The exciting thing for patients with mutations in the GLP-system is that there are FDA-approved medications on the market that mimic the effect of GLP-1. I theorized that these medications may be able to compensate for the low levels of GLP-1 found in these patients, so I offered it as a treatment option to several patients who had failed traditional treatment options and saw excellent results.

The problem is that GLP-1 medications are approved for Type II diabetes and weight loss. If a patient has Type II diabetes, then the process is fairly straightforward, but this is frequently not the case. Many, but not all patients with bulimia nervosa, do qualify for weight loss medications. But weight loss medications in the United States are not required to be covered by insurance plans, so again, this limits access to the medications. Most patients I treat for bulimia either do not have Type II diabetes or do not have coverage for weight loss medications. I have tried on several occasions to make requests for coverage by submitting a 'prior authorization' or by speaking with the Medical Director of a health insurance plan (on the rare occasion a Director will even speak to me), but with limited success. Most insurance companies have no idea how to evaluate whole exome sequencing results and are only required to pay for approved treatments. There is simply no mechanism in place to classify individual disorders or to get coverage for potential treatments.

Chapter 10: The Road Ahead

Imagine all the decisions that you decide to make around food. How would you answer if I asked you to describe all the choices you make about when to eat, what to eat, and when to stop eating? Most people would start by saying that they eat when they are hungry. By this, they typically are referring to times when they have either not eaten in a while or have been very active physically such that they are using more calories. Indeed, energy balance (the need to balance calorie intake with energy expenditure) is a strong driver of hunger, but there are many other factors that go into hunger. We have already touched on one of them— time of day. Circadian rhythms are powerful drivers of appetite, with most people preferring to consume their calories during the daytime. But there are many more factors that influence appetite which we have not yet discussed:

- Thirst— Water balance and food intake are tightly linked. Intake of nutrients can affect the concentration of electrolytes in your blood, and water is used in the metabolism of food. Being dehydrated is a powerful appetite suppressant in most people.

- Inflammation- Most people lose their appetite when they are sick or have a chronic illness like cancer. This occurs because chemical messengers released by immune system cells called cytokines, which cause inflammation, are powerful appetite suppressants.

- GI function— Bloating, constipation or diarrhea, cramping, nausea, and gastroesophageal reflux disorder (also referred to as GERD) can all decrease your desire to eat. We are also just beginning to learn how gut bacteria affect the digestion and absorption of nutrients which can then influence appetite.

• Menstrual cycle— Hormone fluctuations during a woman's normal menstrual cycle can influence appetite, with a higher urge to binge reported during the premenstrual phase.

• Social context— Depending on the situation, you may decide to eat more or less than you normally would. Food is an integral part of many social gatherings, so you may feel more compelled to eat at a holiday, birthday, or dinner party, for instance.

• Availability— Some people are much more likely to eat food when it is free. During medical school and psychiatry residency, I can remember eating more than I normally would when I was on call doing a 30-hour shift, because you never knew when you would be able to eat again.

• Satiation— <u>Satiation</u> refers to how long a certain food will keep you full before you feel hungry again. Certain foods are more filling and influence the timing of meals and snacks.

• Boredom— Many people describe eating as a way of dealing with boredom, even if they are not hungry.

There are also factors that influence *what* you decide to eat:

• Macronutrients— People will often report a different level of desire to eat certain macronutrients, like carbohydrates (sweets) vs. savory foods (fats). Many women report an increased interest in red meat during their period, possibly due to blood loss.

- Cost— Just like people are more likely to eat free food, the cost of food may affect your preferences. Someone may choose to eat a less desirable option because there is less cost involved.

- Appearance— People are more likely to eat food that is more appealing or attractive. You might also eat a food that is novel to you to see what it tastes like.

- Effort— How hard are you willing to work to get a specific type of food? Going to get ice cream may sound good unless you are in the middle of a blizzard and the effort of driving through the snow and ice is not worth the reward of the ice cream.

- Allergies/intolerances— This one is fairly obvious; you are less likely to eat food that makes you sick.

- Fear of choking or vomiting— This is another common concern that many people think about. Many times, a patient will have a bad experience from a food that made them choke or vomit. They will start by avoiding that food, but then keep expanding to cut out more and more things that remind them of the original food that they choked on until they are down to only a few "safe" foods.

Finally, there are factors that influence *how much* you eat:

- Sensory information— Beyond the obvious taste of the food on the tongue, consuming food involves a variety of sensory information, including sound (hearing food being prepared), sight (seeing the food presented), smell, touch (texture), and temperature (hot, cold, spicy). Stretch receptors in your gastrointestinal tract also send signals that the muscles in your stomach are expanding to hold the food and that you are literally 'full'.

● Hormones— There are several hormones that are released after you eat to help you digest, absorb, and store food. Many of these hormones also send signals back to the brain to tell you to stop eating. We have already touched on a few of these in the book, including insulin and glucagon-like peptide 1, but there are several others, including cholecystokinin, protein YY, and gastric inhibitory polypeptide.

● Others— Just like social setting, cost, and palatability can influence *when* you decide to eat, they can also influence *how much* you eat. Indulging may be more acceptable during certain celebrations, while many people do not feel comfortable eating in front of others and may choose to eat less than they normally would for fear of judgment.

This list is by no means comprehensive, but it does give you an idea of how complex the decision to eat and drink can be. Food and water are essential to survive, but they can also kill you due to food-borne illnesses, so it makes sense that the body has complex systems to decide when, what, and how much to eat. I can think of patients who have had issues in every one of these areas (whether it is genetic, psychological, or social). Right now, clinicians only measure a fraction of these things when a patient comes in with a concern about eating. When someone comes in underweight (whether it is anorexia nervosa or avoidant restrictive food intake disorder), the standard treatment is essentially to put the patient on a high calorie diet and use coping skills and medications to help them tolerate the distress of doing something that the patient hates. For patients with binge eating disorder or bulimia nervosa, clinicians use a combination of medications to reduce binging behaviors (like stimulants or antidepressants) and teach coping skills the patient can use instead of binging or purging when they feel stressed.

Now imagine an alternative world in which a patient can come in with their concerns about eating and, in addition to whole exome sequencing, we can get a more complete picture of what may be contributing to their problems:

- *Bioinformatics*— Bioinformatics broadly refers to the use of computer programs to analyze large sets of biological data. Clinicians can already sequence a person's DNA to identify all the mutations that may affect their metabolism, hormones, or neurotransmitters, but there are limitations in being able to determine which mutations actually change how a protein functions and which have no effect. There are several programs that are available now that do predict if a mutation is damaging or tolerated, but they, too, have limitations. These programs are not able to factor in the consequences of other mutations within the same gene or mutations in the other copy of the same gene. They also are not able to factor in a series of mutations in genes in the same pathway. For example, I had a patient with two mutations in the genes involved in the two final steps of cholesterol synthesis. Each mutation was predicted to have a modest effect on the function of each protein, but what is the combined effect of the two mutations? Another smaller problem is that most mutations either have no effect on the function of a protein, or damage its functioning, but there are some mutations that make it work more effectively. These mutations are called gain-of-function or increase-of-function mutations and have the complete opposite effect of what you might predict. Being able to identify the occasional gain-of-function mutation could be incredibly helpful.

• *Metabolomics*— <u>Metabolomics</u> is an intimidating word, but it is essentially the study of all the chemical processes in the body. It is now possible to measure a wide variety of molecules important to the functioning of the body, including lipids, carbohydrates, amino acids, nucleotides, and products resulting from synthesizing or breaking down these compounds[144]. I have presented in this book the theory that some cases of anorexia nervosa are the result of impairments in converting nutrients like fatty acids and amino acids into energy, and that the buildup of these nutrients is what triggers the aversion to food. Companies like Genova Diagnostics are now able to measure the levels

of these molecules using their NutrEval® testing to determine if there is in fact a buildup of nutrients that the body has a hard time metabolizing. Combining DNA sequencing with metabolomics may better identify these back-ups in the system and allow for the design of specific treatments to work around these blockades.

• *Gut health*— There has already been a tremendous effort to explore the role of gut health, including gut bacteria or the <u>microbiome</u>, in eating disorders. Imagine being able to measure digestive efficiency (the amount of nutrients that the body can extract from food before it is passed along as waste), and gut motility (how well the gut moves food through the gastrointestinal tract). I have many patients with mutations in genes related to the digestion and absorption of fat that report oily or bulky stools. These patients are often placed on extremely high meals plans in order to restore weight. Sadly, this inability to restore weight is often used against a patient as evidence that they don't want to get better or are actively undermining their treatment. Clinicians may soon be able to identify which nutrients a patient has a hard time digesting and absorbing and design specific meal plans for them, or correct imbalances in gut bacteria that could be contributing to their problems.

• *Wearable devices*— Wearable devices offer hope for gathering dramatically more useful information than I can get in a one-hour appointment in my office. Watches can monitor physical activity, estimate the amount of sleep and the number of times someone wakes up through the night, and determine circadian rhythms. Devices that measure body temperature and glucose levels and monitor heart rate are also available. Most of these devices collect measurements continuously 24 hours a day for several days. Clinicians may soon be able to predict things like when a patient is starting to binge eat, is slipping into a manic phase, or has developed a sleep disorder.

In the future, clinicians will be able to get a complete picture of a patient's functioning, including their genetics, metabolism, microbiome, and circadian rhythms. With this information, clinicians will be able to formulate individual plans for nutrition, vitamins/supplements, daily activity, and (if needed) medications instead of relying on the one-size-fits-all approach currently offered by treatment programs. This is the future that I imagined when I first set out to find "something better."

To learn more about GIFTED and Dr Lutter visit:

<u>www.Precision-Psychiatry.com</u>[1]

[1] https://www.who.int/news-room/fact-sheets/detail/depression

[2] https://psychiatry.org/psychiatrists/practice/dsm/about-dsm/history-of-the-dsm

[3] https://ps.psychiatryonline.org/doi/10.1176/ps.51.1.41

[4] https://psychmuseum.uwgb.org/clinical/dsm/

[5] https://psychiatry.org/psychiatrists/practice/dsm/about-dsm/history-of-the-dsm

[6] https://www.mdpi.com/2076-328X/6/1/5

[7]   https://slate.com/technology/2013/04/diagnostic-and-statistical-manual-fifth-edition-why-will-half-the-u-s-population-have-a-mental-illness.html

[8] Ironically neither Alcohol Abuse or Alcoholism is an official diagnosis anymore in DSM-V (https://www.niaaa.nih.gov/publications/brochures-and-fact-sheets/alcohol-use-disorder-comparison-between-dsm). Perhaps they should change their name to the National Institute of Alcohol Use Disorders or NIAUD to keep up with the times.

[9] https://www.ncbi.nlm.nih.gov/pmc/articles/PMC4724794/

[10]   https://www.theguardian.com/society/2016/jan/27/prozac-next-psychiatric-wonder-drug-research-medicine-mental-illness

[11] https://bpspubs.onlinelibrary.wiley.com/doi/full/10.1111/bcp.14327

[12] https://www.nimh.nih.gov/funding/grant-writing-and-application-process/peer-review-committees

[13] https://report.nih.gov/nihdatabook/category/10

---

1. http://www.precision-psychiatry.com/

[14] https://www.vox.com/the-highlight/2019/6/3/18271538/open-access-elsevier-california-sci-hub-academic-paywalls

[15] https://tidsskriftet.no/en/2020/08/kronikk/money-behind-academic-publishing

[16] https://www.investors.com/etfs-and-funds/sectors/sp500-most-profitable-u-s-companies-practically-print-money/

[17] https://www.ncbi.nlm.nih.gov/pmc/articles/PMC3809805/

[18] https://www.theguardian.com/science/2021/may/21/research-findings-that-are-probably-wrong-cited-far-more-than-robust-ones-study-finds

[19] https://www.nature.com/articles/d41586-019-02479-7

[20] https://www.nature.com/articles/d41586-019-02479-7

[21] https://www.pnas.org/doi/10.1073/pnas.0508901103

[22] https://www.nature.com/articles/nature10907

[23] https://rettsyndrome.wordpress.com/tag/bone-marrow-transplant/

[24] https://www.nature.com/articles/nature14444#Sec4

[25] https://www.sciencenews.org/article/cancer-biology-studies-research-replication-reproducibility

[26] https://www.psychreg.org/replication-crisis-psychology/

[27] https://www.science.org/content/article/potential-fabrication-research-images-threatens-key-theory-alzheimers-disease

[28] verywellmind.com/wait-list-control-group-1067234

[29] https://www.ncbi.nlm.nih.gov/pmc/articles/PMC6493527/

[30] https://www.ncbi.nlm.nih.gov/pmc/articles/PMC5033643/

[31] https://www.thennt.com/nnt/vitamin-d-for-fracture-prevention-elderly-nursing-home/

[32] https://psychnews.psychiatryonline.org/doi/10.1176/appi.pn.2018.8b20

[33] In theory pharmaceutical companies can no longer bury negative findings, because every study must be registered with a database called ClinicalTrials.gov before starting if it wants to be published. In practice, every few clinicians know of the existence of this database, let alone how to search it and interpret the results of an unpublished study.

[34] The one exception to this is Clinical Psychology doctorate programs which tend to provide very rigorous training in both.

[35] https://journals.lww.com/hrpjournal/Abstract/2003/03000/_On_Cyclic_Insanity__by_Karl_Ludwig_Kahlbaum,_MD_.3.aspx

[36] http://ids-qids.org/

[37] https://www.gatewaypsychiatric.com/rdocs-and-dsm-5-diagnosis-and-psychiatry/

[38] negative valence, positive valence, social processes, arousal and regulatory systems, and sensorimotor systems

[39] https://www.nimh.nih.gov/about/director/messages/2017/the-future-of-rdoc

[40] https://www.optum.com/business/insights/pharmacy-care-services/page.hub.high-cost-gene-therapies.html

[41] The exception of those on the X and Y sex chromosomes – biological females have two copies of all X-linked genes and no Y-linked genes, and biological males have one copy of each X- and Y-linked gene

[42] https://obamawhitehouse.archives.gov/blog/2015/01/30/precision-medicine-initiative-data-driven-treatments-unique-your-own-body

[43] https://medlineplus.gov/genetics/understanding/precisionmedicine/definition/

[44] https://hdsr.mitpress.mit.edu/pub/y7r65r4k/release/4

[45] https://ascopubs.org/doi/full/10.1200/EDBK_174176

[46] https://www.nejm.org/doi/full/10.1056/nejmp1500523

[47] https://pubmed.ncbi.nlm.nih.gov/28403846/

[48] https://www.precisionmedicine.columbia.edu/content/precision-psychiatry

[49] https://www.massgeneral.org/psychiatry/research/precision-psychiatry

[50] https://www.stanfordpmhw.com/

[51] https://mghcme.org/precision2022/

[52] https://www.appi.org/Products/Neuropsychiatry-and-Biological-Psychiatry/Precision-Psychiatry

[53] https://www.psychiatrictimes.com/view/psychiatric-pharmacogenomic-testing-evidence-base

[54] https://pubmed.ncbi.nlm.nih.gov/28403846/

[55] https://pubmed.ncbi.nlm.nih.gov/36274532/

[56] Baselmans, B.M.L, et al. Biol Psychiatry. 2021 Jan 1;89(1):11-19.

[57] https://journals.plos.org/plosone/article?id=10.1371/journal.pone.0181556

[58] https://link.springer.com/article/10.1007/s10989-021-10309-6

[59] https://pubmed.ncbi.nlm.nih.gov/33396962/

[60] https://www.frontiersin.org/articles/10.3389/fpsyt.2015.00105/full

[61] https://pubmed.ncbi.nlm.nih.gov/35396579/

[62] https://www.frontiersin.org/articles/10.3389/fgene.2018.00406/full

[63] https://pubmed.ncbi.nlm.nih.gov/34183866/

[64] https://pubmed.ncbi.nlm.nih.gov/35396579/

[65] https://www.breastcancer.org/risk/risk-factors/genetics

[66] https://gnomad.broadinstitute.org/gene/ENSG00000012048?dataset=gnomad_r2_1

[67] https://www.breastcancer.org/facts-statistics

[68] https://www.psychiatry.org/psychiatrists/practice/dsm

[69] the most common form of purging is self-induced vomiting but actually encompasses a large range of behaviors including laxative abuse, misuse of medications like thyroid medications, or use drugs to suppress appetite

[70] excessive exercise is not considered a purging behavior in this case

[71] Called carnitine palmitoyltransferase 1 and 2

[72] which can stand for either mammalian target of rapamycin or mechanistic target of rapamycin

[73] https://www.ncbi.nlm.nih.gov/pmc/articles/PMC5391759/

[74] https://www.ncbi.nlm.nih.gov/pmc/articles/PMC4935144/

[75] https://pubmed.ncbi.nlm.nih.gov/34419970/

[76] https://pubmed.ncbi.nlm.nih.gov/21982706/

[77] https://pubmed.ncbi.nlm.nih.gov/29914932/

[78] https://pubmed.ncbi.nlm.nih.gov/3164990/

[79] https://pubmed.ncbi.nlm.nih.gov/30981752/

[80] https://pubmed.ncbi.nlm.nih.gov/15569892/

[81] https://pubmed.ncbi.nlm.nih.gov/8191873/

[82] https://pubmed.ncbi.nlm.nih.gov/17117412/

[83] https://pubmed.ncbi.nlm.nih.gov/35850019/

[84] https://www.mdpi.com/1422-0067/21/5/1642/htm

[85] https://pubmed.ncbi.nlm.nih.gov/34225929/

[86] My theory is that a lot of this food simply comes out of their feces without being absorbed as many people will tell me that their stools are bulky and oily, but I have not tested this theory yet. It is possible to measure the amount of unabsorbed energy in mice by literally burning their poop and measuring the amount of heat produced in something called a Bomb Calorimeter, but alas this technique is only available for research studies and not clinical care.

[87] https://health.clevelandclinic.org/do-i-need-to-worry-about-eating-complete-proteins/

[88] Charts are published by the Centers for Disease Control that show the normal growth trajectories of boys and girls from birth to 18 years of age. There are lines that the 5% (that is 95% of people the same age are taller or weigh more), 10%, 25%, 50%, 75%, 90% and 95% (that is individuals who are taller or weigh more than 95% of all other people the same age).

[89] https://www.sciencedirect.com/science/article/abs/pii/S1051227606000148

[90] Endorphins are often credited for the 'runner's high that comes with exercise.' While it is true that endorphins increase with exercise, it is not clear that it is the actual cause of the euphoria (endogenous (endogenous meaning inner or produced by the body)

[91] Indeed, it is the very presence of the endogenous opioids that allow for the existence of the exogenous opioids. Drugs like heroin act like beta-endorphin but are much, much more powerful in essence hi-jacking the system.

[92] The mutation is labeled as rs28942372

[93] Opioid receptors are highly expressed in the gut and slow down movement of food through the gastrointestinal tract. The anti-diarrheal medication loperamide acts in the opioid system and constipation is a well-known consequence of addiction to painkillers like oxycodone.

[94] https://gnomad.broadinstitute.org/variant/2-25384048-G-C?dataset=gnomad_r2_1

[95] Possibly because while it does decrease beta-endorphin levels it also creates a new neuropeptide with beta-endorphin attached to the end of beta-melanocyte stimulating hormone. Beta-melanocyte stimulating hormone also affects appetite and it is not clear what are the consequences of attaching beta-endorphin to beta-melanocyte stimulating hormone.

[96] https://journals.plos.org/plosone/article?id=10.1371/journal.pone.0181556

[97] Mol Metab 2013; 2:423–434.

[98] Cell Rep. 2017 Aug 22;20(8):1881-1892.

[99] https://pubmed.ncbi.nlm.nih.gov/22800867/

[100] https://pubmed.ncbi.nlm.nih.gov/27030669/

[101] There are at least 14 different serotonin receptors grouped into 7 families: https://en.wikipedia.org/wiki/5-HT_receptor

[102] Tetrahydrobiopterin is also involved in making a molecule called nitric oxide which causes blood vessels to dilate and in breaking down the amino acid phenylalanine. Inability to break down phenylalanine causes a rare neurological disorder called phenylketonuria.

[103] The word circadian is derived from Greek. Circa- about and dia- day referring to anything that is about a day long.

[104] https://pubmed.ncbi.nlm.nih.gov/24216484/

[105] https://pubmed.ncbi.nlm.nih.gov/9989497/

[106] https://www.frontiersin.org/articles/10.3389/fphys.2019.00682/full

[107] https://www.verywellhealth.com/zeitgebers-and-how-they-work-3015395

[108] Carbohydrates are the preferred energy source for the brain and prolonged periods of sleep deprivation are often accompanied by intense cravings for sweets, which is probably due to the increased energy required for consciousness.

[109] https://www.ncbi.nlm.nih.gov/pmc/articles/PMC3136184/

[110] https://my.clevelandclinic.org/health/diseases/21665-cannabis-hyperemesis-syndrome

[111] PLoS One. 2015; 10(11): e0140592.

[112] Diabetologia. 2010;53(12):2629–40. 10.1007/s00125-010-

[113] https://www.healthline.com/health/food-nutrition/benefits-vitamin-d

[114] Neurol Ther. 2018 Jun;7(1):59-85. doi: 10.1007/s40120-017-0086-4. Epub 2017 Dec 14.

[115] Rev Neurosci. 2017 Feb 1;28(2):185-201. doi: 10.1515/revneuro-2016-0044.

[116] Diabetes. 2008 Oct;57(10):2569-76

[117] Diabetes. 2001 Jan;50(1):105-12.

[118] Science. 2022 Feb 25;375(6583):

[119] In this section I will focus on biologically active molecules including medications, vitamins, and supplements as I am not an expert in other forms of treatment like neurostimulation or developing new forms of psychotherapy.

[120] https://www.ehealthinsurance.com/medicare/coverage/medicare-part-d-brand-name-vs-generic-drugs/

[121] https://www.sofpromed.com/how-much-does-a-clinical-trial-cost

[122] https://www.fiercepharma.com/sales-and-marketing/updated-shire-s-vyvanse-brand-team-draws-fire-for-aggressive-binge-eating-push

[123] https://medlineplus.gov/druginfo/meds/a682245.html

[124] https://pubmed.ncbi.nlm.nih.gov/10732660/

[125] https://pubmed.ncbi.nlm.nih.gov/27828694/

[126] https://pubmed.ncbi.nlm.nih.gov/27930498/

[127] A medication used to prevent pain during surgeries or medical procedures.

[128] https://www.ncbi.nlm.nih.gov/pmc/articles/PMC5126726/

[129] https://pubmed.ncbi.nlm.nih.gov/16894061/

[130] https://www.greenbrooktms.com/blog/the-history-of-antidepressants

[131] https://pubmed.ncbi.nlm.nih.gov/35451097/

[132] https://pubmed.ncbi.nlm.nih.gov/35977629/

[133] https://pubmed.ncbi.nlm.nih.gov/33022440/

[134] https://www.reuters.com/article/us-johnson-johnson-fda-pricing/jj-prices-ketamine-like-depression-treatment-at-590-885-for-two-doses-idUSKCN1QN2AX

[135] https://www.accessdata.fda.gov/drugsatfda_docs/label/2017/021083s059,021110s076lbl.pdf

[136] https://pubmed.ncbi.nlm.nih.gov/36462440/

[137] https://pubmed.ncbi.nlm.nih.gov/35429726/

[138] https://www.ncbi.nlm.nih.gov/pmc/articles/PMC6909887/

[139] https://pubmed.ncbi.nlm.nih.gov/32092760/

[140] https://medlineplus.gov/druginfo/meds/a602026.html

[141] https://pubmed.ncbi.nlm.nih.gov/34836413/

[142] https://pubmed.ncbi.nlm.nih.gov/35326338/

[143] https://pubmed.ncbi.nlm.nih.gov/35997954/

[144] Cold Spring Harb Mol Case Stud. 2015 Oct; 1(1): a000588.

www.ingramcontent.com/pod-product-compliance
Lightning Source LLC
Chambersburg PA
CBHW060929140726
47996CB00001B/432